Workbook to Accompany

Body Structures & Functions

10th Edition

Ann Senisi Scott

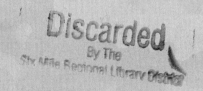
07-2143

THOMSON
—
DELMAR LEARNING   Australia   Canada   Mexico   Singapore   Spain   United Kingdom   United States

THOMSON
*
DELMAR LEARNING™

Workbook to Accompany Body Structures & Functions, 10th Edition
by Ann Senisi Scott

Vice President, Health Care Business Unit
William Brottmiller

Editorial Director
Cathy L. Esperti

Acquisitions Editor
Sherry Gomoll

Developmental Editor
Darcy M. Scelsi

Editorial Assistant
Jennifer Conklin

Marketing Director
Jennifer McAvey

Project Editor
Shelley Esposito

Production Editor
John Mickelbank

Art and Design Coordinator
Robert Plante

ISBN 1-4018-0997-9

Library of Congress Cataloging-in-Publication Number
2004031519

NOTICE TO THE READER

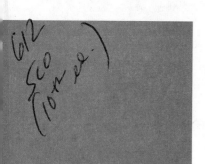

CONTENTS

Introduction to the Structural Units

OVERVIEW

This chapter is an introduction to the study of the *structure* (anatomy) and *function* (physiology) of the body.

Anatomic Terminology

Anatomy and physiology have their own terminology to describe the parts of the body and their location or position.

In the anatomical position, the body is erect, the person is facing forward with arms at his or her sides, the palms are outward, and the feet are parallel.

Branches of anatomy subdivide the field depending on the information needed:

Gross anatomy can be seen by the naked eye.

Microscopic anatomy is seen by the microscope.

Developmental anatomy is the study of the body from its beginning and through its lifetime.

Comparative anatomy compares human anatomy with animal anatomy.

Systematic anatomy is the study of the body organs that make up a system.

Terms that refer to the location and direction of the body usually are described in pairs:

Anterior (ventral): front / posterior (dorsal): back
Cranial: toward the head or top / caudal: toward the tail or bottom
Superior: above another part / inferior: below another part
Medial: toward the middle / lateral: toward the side
Proximal: close to the point of attachment / distal: away from the point of attachment
Superficial (external): at the surface of the body / deep (internal): deeper in the body

Body planes are imaginary dividing lines to help separate the body: *sagittal* (right and left sections), *coronal* and *ventral* (anterior and posterior portions), and *transverse* (upper and lower parts).

The organs of the body are located in cavities. The terms used to describe the body cavities are:

Dorsal: posterior, includes cranial and spinal cavities

Ventral: anterior, includes thoracic and abdominopelvic cavities

Another way of describing where the abdominopelvic organs are located is by one of the following nine regions: epigastric, right and left hypochondriac, umbilical, right and left lumbar, hypogastric, and right and left iliac (inguinal) areas.

Life Functions

Life functions are the necessary activities that allow living organs to grow and function. These activities include movement, ingestion, digestion, transport, respiration, synthesis, assimilation, growth, secretion, excretion, regulation, and reproduction.

Body processes include metabolism. **Metabolism** consists of two processes, *anabolism* and *catabolism*. Cell functioning requires a stable cellular environment; maintaining this process is known as *homeostasis.*

ACTIVITIES

A. Use the words in the following list to complete the statements. Terms are used only once.

anatomy   gross anatomy

biology   histology

cytology   microscopic anatomy

dermatology   neurology

embryology   physiology

endocrinology   systematic anatomy

1. The study of all life forms is _____.

2. Through the study of _____ _____, we can extend the knowledge of body parts.

3. A study of blood tissue is called _____.

4. The study of the nervous system is called _____.

5. _____ _____ is the study of the organs that make up parts of the organ system.

6. _____ is the study of how our organs function.

7. The study of the cells is called _____.

8. The study of human cells from fertilization to birth is called _____.

9. The study of the size and shape of an organ is called _____.

10. _____ is the study of the hormonal system.

B. Anatomy is subdivided into many branches based on the type of knowledge sought. Identify the branch of anatomy that is described in the following statements.

1. The study of the structure and function of various organs or parts making up a particular organ system is _____.

2. The study of the growth and development of an organism during its lifetime is

   _____.

3. The study of anatomy at the microscopic level that is further divided into cytology and histology is _____.

4. The study of the different body parts and organs of humans with regard to similarities and differences of other animals in the animal kingdom is _____.

5. The study of large and easily observable structures on an organism is

   _____.

C. Select the letter of the choice that best completes the statement.

1. The body in the anatomical position is:
   a. standing erect, face forward, arms at the sides, palms forward, feet parallel
   b. standing erect, face forward, arms at the back, palms forward, feet parallel
   c. standing erect, face forward, arms at the front, palms forward, feet parallel
   d. standing erect, face forward, arms at the sides, palms backward, feet parallel

2. The vertical cut that divides the body into anterior and posterior sections is called the:
   a. horizontal plane
   b. sagittal plane
   c. transverse plane
   d. coronal plane

3. The horizontal cut dividing the body into upper and lower sections is called the:
   a. frontal plane
   b. transverse plane
   c. sagittal plane
   d. coronal plane

4. An imaginary dividing line useful in separating the body is a:
   a. section
   b. cavity
   c. quadrant
   d. plane

5. The lacrimal ducts are located in the:
   a. oral cavity
   b. buccal cavity
   c. orbital cavity
   d. otic cavity

6. The formation and release of substance from a cell or structure is called:
   a. assimilation
   b. excretion
   c. secretion
   d. synthesis

7. The oxidation of food molecules is called:
   a. regulation
   b. respiration
   c. reproduction
   d. secretion

8. Combination of simple molecules into more complex units to build new tissue is:
   a. digestion
   b. ingestion
   c. regulation
   d. synthesis

9. The building up and breaking down of cell material is called:
   a. catabolism
   b. anabolism
   c. metabolism
   d. homeostasis

10. Maintenance of optimum cell functioning requires a balanced cell environment called:
    a. regulation
    b. homeostasis
    c. metabolism
    d. catabolism

D. Label the two diagrams on this page.

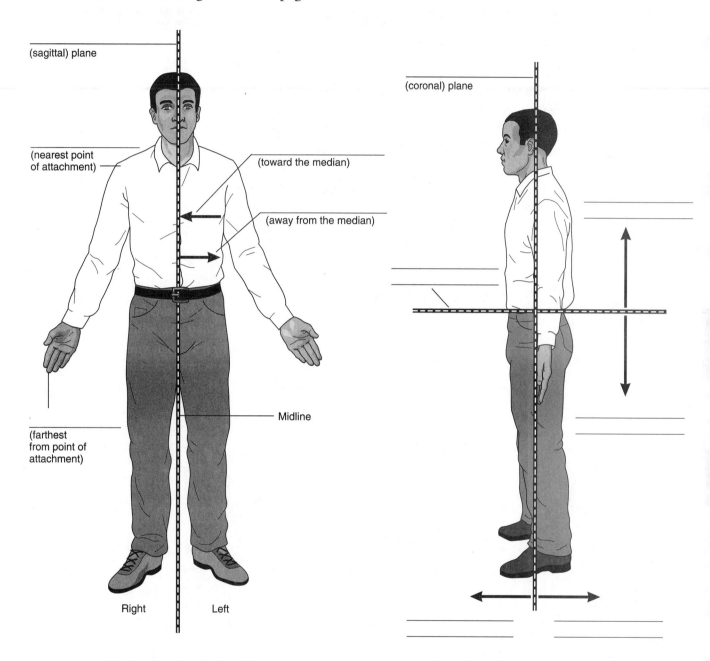

(sagittal) plane

(nearest point of attachment)

(toward the median)

(away from the median)

(farthest from point of attachment)

Midline

Right   Left

(coronal) plane

Anatomical terms used to describe body division into parts

Imaginary lines, or planes, separate body structures

E. Match the letters in Column B with the most appropriate term in Column A.

Column A	Column B
_____ 1. brain	a. spinal cavity
_____ 2. bronchi	b. abdominal cavity
_____ 3. hypogastric region	c. region just below the sternum
_____ 4. urinary bladder	d. orbital cavity
_____ 5. stomach	e. pelvic cavity
_____ 6. mediastinum	f. pubic areas
_____ 7. epigastric region	g. midpoint of thoracic cavity
_____ 8. heart	h. pericardial cavity
_____ 9. vertebrae	i. thoracic cavity
_____ 10. eyes	j. cranial cavity

F. Label the cavities of the body: Color the posterior brown, the anterior yellow, the thoracic green, and the abdominopelvic blue.

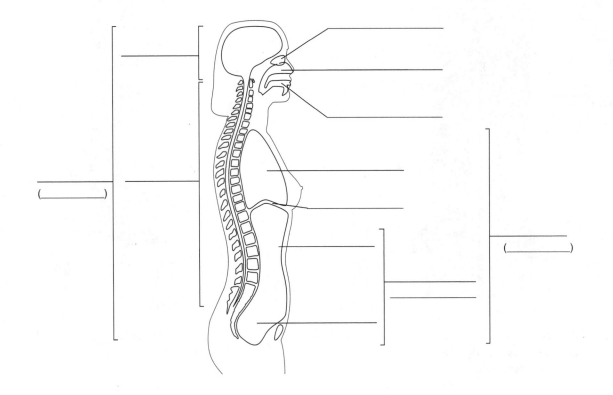

G. Match the number on the abdominal region with the correct description.

_____ right hypochondriac

_____ epigastric

_____ left hypochondriac

_____ right lumbar

_____ umbilical

_____ left lumbar

_____ right iliac

_____ hypogastric

_____ left iliac

H. Circle the mismatched pairs.

1. Superior/inferior

2. Secretion/endocrine system

3. Teeth/orbital cavity

4. Movement/respiratory system

5. Proximal/distal

6. Medial/lateral

7. Caudal/posterior

8. Anterior/ventral

I. Fill in the blanks to complete the statements on body processes.

The functional activities that result in growth and repair of body tissue are called _____. This function consists of two processes that have opposite effects, namely _____ and _____. The taking in of food and oxygen occurs in the _____ state which builds up _____ materials from simpler ones. The release of energy and carbon dioxide occurs in the _____ state which is the breaking down of _____ substances into simpler ones. These functions require a stable, _____ environment; maintaining this internal environment is known as _____.

J. Fill in the blanks relating to body planes from the following word list:

anterior   posterior

distal   proximal

inferior   superior

In the study of body parts and planes,
you need to describe the place or part by name.

If you look at the trunk it is _____.
If the buttocks are in view it is _____.

If the location is _____ it is above a certain part,
while the navel is _____ to the heart.

The wrist is _____ to the shoulder joint,
while the elbow is _____ to the shoulder attachment point.

Is it superficial or internal? You must know!
Or is medial or lateral the way to go?

When all is said and done,
anatomical directions can be fun.

APPLYING THEORY TO PRACTICE

1. You are directed to an anatomical model to place the organs in the correct body cavity. Name the cavity in which you would place the following:

esophagus	_____	nose	_____
pancreas	_____	eyes	_____
appendix	_____	small intestine	_____
heart	_____	mouth	_____
spinal cord	_____	reproductive organs	_____
ribs	_____	lungs	_____
urinary bladder	_____	liver	_____
brain	_____	trachea	_____

2. Think about the following activities occurring within your body at this moment. These activities include movement, digestion, respiration, secretion, and transport. What is their function to your well-being?

Movement: _____

_____

Digestion: _____

_____

Respiration: _____

_____

Secretion: _____

_____

Transport: _____

_____

3. As a medical assistant in a doctor's office you must know medical terminology. Use the correct term for the region or location to describe the following situations.

a. Mr. David is a construction worker who comes to the office with severe pain in his back. The pain is located in the _____.

b. Mrs. Andrews, age 55, is scheduled to have gallbladder surgery. She wants to know where she may have a scar. _____

c. Kenneth is complaining of severe pains in his stomach. Where is the pain located?

_____

d. Leslie comes to the office complaining of having severe menstrual cramps over the last 4 months. The pain is located in the _____.

e. Jimmy, age 4, fell while playing and has an abrasion on the lower part of his right arm. The area of the abrasion is located _____ to the elbow.

KRISS KROSS PUZZLE

The words are listed in alphabetical order according to length. Fit them into their proper places in the Kriss Kross. The words refer to anatomical terminology.

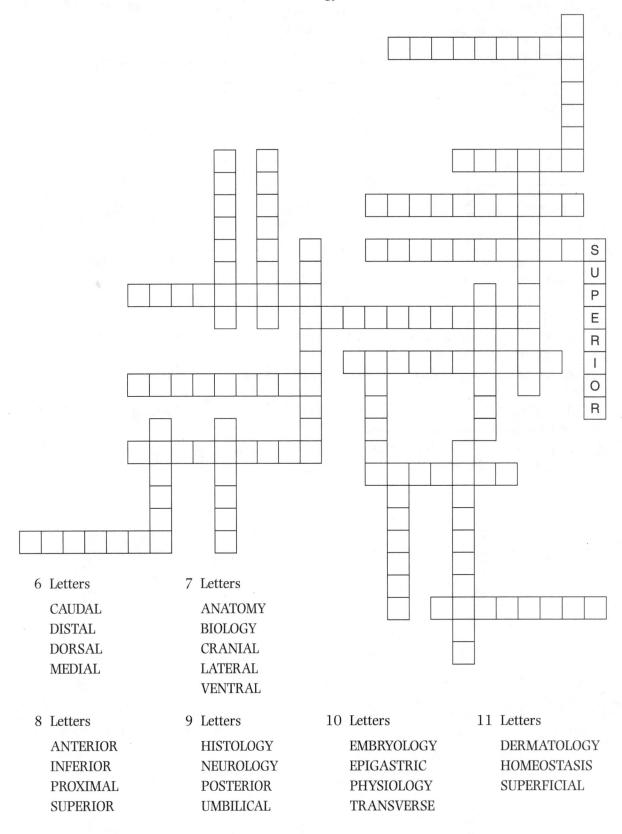

6 Letters	7 Letters
CAUDAL	ANATOMY
DISTAL	BIOLOGY
DORSAL	CRANIAL
MEDIAL	LATERAL
	VENTRAL

8 Letters	9 Letters	10 Letters	11 Letters
ANTERIOR	HISTOLOGY	EMBRYOLOGY	DERMATOLOGY
INFERIOR	NEUROLOGY	EPIGASTRIC	HOMEOSTASIS
PROXIMAL	POSTERIOR	PHYSIOLOGY	SUPERFICIAL
SUPERIOR	UMBILICAL	TRANSVERSE	

SURF THE NET

Briefly summarize your findings from the suggested Web sites or alternate sites. Follow the instructions at the suggested sites.

1. To understand how the body is divided into planes and sections go to:
   http://www.madsci.org/~lynn/VH/planes.html

2. To review the body cavities and participate in an interactive quiz go to:
   http://www.gen.umn.edu/faculty_staff/jensen/1135/webanatomy

3. To understand how the body maintains its internal structure environment through negative feedback to to:
   http://www.ecsu.ctsateu.edu/personal/faculty/saull/sect9/resous9/cartoons9/homeos9/html

Chapter 2

Chemistry of Living Things

OVERVIEW

Chemistry is the study of the structure of matter. **Matter** is anything that has weight and occupies space. **Energy** is the ability to do work; it can be potential or kinetic energy.

An **atom** is the smallest piece of an element. It is made of subatomic particles; namely, *protons, neutrons,* and *electrons.* The number of protons and neutrons is equal in the nucleus of the atom. **Isotopes** are atoms of a specific element that have the same number of protons but a different number of neutrons in their nuclei.

Elements are formed from atoms that are alike. **Compounds** are elements that combine in a definite proportion by weight. The smallest unit of a compound is a **molecule.**

Ions are the smallest particles of a molecule and have a positive or negative charge. When compounds are in solution and act as if they have broken into individual pieces (ions), the elements of the compound are **electrolytes.**

Compounds

Types of compounds are *inorganic* and *organic.* Inorganic compounds do not usually contain carbon; water is the most important inorganic compound. Organic compounds always contain the element carbon. The four main groups of organic compounds are *carbohydrates, lipids, proteins,* and *nucleic acids.*

Carbohydrates consist of carbon, hydrogen, and oxygen. They are subdivided into monosaccharide, disaccharide, and polysaccharide.

Lipids are made of carbon, hydrogen, and oxygen; they differ from carbohydrates, because there is less oxygen in relation to hydrogen.

Proteins contain carbon, hydrogen, oxygen, and nitrogen, and usually some phosphorous and sulfur. *Enzymes* are specialized proteins that help control the various chemical reactions occurring in the cell; they act as catalysts.

Nucleic acids are organic compounds containing carbon, hydrogen, oxygen, nitrogen, and phosphorous; the two most important are deoxyribonucleic acid (DNA) and ribonucleic acid (RNA).

Acids, Bases, and Salts

Acids, bases, and **salts** are organic and inorganic compounds found in living organisms. An acid is a substance that when dissolved in water will ionize into positively charged hydrogen ions. A base or alkali is a substance that when dissolved in water ionizes into negatively charged hydroxide ions. When an acid and base combine they form a *salt* and *water*. This reaction is called *neutralization*.

The pH Scale

To measure the acidity or alkalinity of a solution, a **pH scale** is used. pH means the potential of hydrogen. A pH of 7 is neutral; it has an equal number of hydrogen and hydroxide ions. A pH between 0 and 6.9 indicates an acidic solution; a pH between 7.1 and 14 indicates an alkaline or basic solution. Water is neutral and has a pH of 7, whereas blood is slightly alkaline, with a pH of 7.35 to 7.45. For living cells to function, their biochemical reactions must maintain homeostasis in their acid-base and electrolyte balance.

Medical Imaging

Nuclear medicine uses radionuclides to scan the body. Types include computerized axial tomography (CAT), positron emission tomography (PET), sonography, and magnetic resonance imaging (MRI). These noninvasive techniques are used for diagnostic purposes.

ACTIVITIES

A. These statements relate to matter and energy. Use the words in the following list to complete the statements.

bone	kinetic energy
created	energy
blood	destroyed
oxygen	physical change
chemical change	potential energy

1. An example of solid matter in the body is _____.

2. Matter can neither be _____ nor _____, it can change form through physical or chemical means.

3. Chewing a piece of toast is an example of a _____ _____ in matter.

4. An example of liquid matter in the body is _____; an example of gaseous matter in the body is _____.

5. Sitting in a chair would be an example of _____ _____.

6. If _____ is the ability to do work, a type of _____ that results in movement or motion would be _____ _____.

B. Select the letter of the choice that best completes the statement.

1. The ability to do work is called:
   a. matter
   b. energy
   c. physical change
   d. chemical change

2. The subatomic particles with a positive (+) charge are called:
   a. neutrons
   b. electrons
   c. protons
   d. atoms

3. The four main groups of organic compounds are:
   a. carbohydrates, lipids, proteins, and DNA
   b. carbohydrates, lipids, proteins, and nucleic acids
   c. carbohydrates, lipids, proteins, and monosaccharides
   d. carbohydrates, lipids, proteins, and RNA

4. Lipids or fats may also be known as all of the following except:
   a. fatty acids
   b. cholesterol
   c. glycogen
   d. triglycerides

5. The reaction that occurs when an acid and base are combined is:
   a. neutralization
   b. dehydration
   c. synthesis
   d. compound

6. Dehydration synthesis involves the synthesis of a large molecule from small ones by:
   a. the addition of a molecule of H_2O
   b. the addition of a molecule of CHO
   c. the loss of a molecule of H_2O
   d. the loss of a molecule of CHO

7. The nitrogenous bases of the rungs of the DNA ladder are paired as follows:
   a. thymine with adenine
   b. thymine with cytosine
   c. thymine with guanine
   d. adenine with cytosine

8. A diagnostic test to determine the effects of a stroke is:
   a. magnetic resonance imaging (MRI)
   b. Doppler scan
   c. computerized axial tomography (CAT)
   d. positron electron emission (PET)

9. Specialized protein molecules that help control cell activity are:
   a. triglycerides
   b. amino acids
   c. enzymes
   d. nucleic acids

10. pH measures the acidity or alkalinity of a solution. A solution with a pH of 8 would be:
    a. neutral
    b. acidic
    c. alkaline
    d. strongly acidic

C. Label the following diagram and color the neutrons, protons, and electrons, using a different color for each.

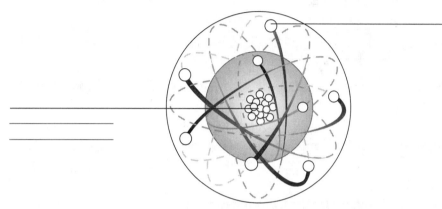

Structure of an atom

D. Answer the following questions.

1. In the previous diagram, how many protons, neutrons, and electrons are illustrated?

   _____

2. When an atom has six protons, six neutrons, and six electrons, is it positive, negative, or neutral?

   _____

3. When atom A gives up an electron to atom B, it now has more protons than electrons. What does this mean?

   _____

4. The atom B that took up the extra electron now has more electrons than protons. What does this mean?

   _____

   _____

5. These charged atoms are now called _____.

6. If an atom has an equal number of protons but a different number of neutrons it is called an

   _____.

7. When an _____ comes apart it gives off energy in what form? How is this used for medical purposes?

   _____

   _____

   _____

E. Circle the correctly spelled word in each of the following statements about elements, compounds, and molecules.

1. Atoms that are alike combine to form elements that can (neither, niether) be (created, crated) nor destroyed.

2. Each element is represented by a (chemicle, chemical) symbol.

3. Elements combine in (porportion, proportion) by (wait, weight) to form compounds.

4. (Separately, separatly), hydrogen and oxygen are gases, and when they unite to form the compound water the substance now has (deferent, different) characteristics.

5. Most living organisms will take the 20 (essential, esential) elements and change them into the compounds needed by the body.

6. The smallest unit of a compound that still has the properties of the compound is called a (molecul, molecule).

7. When compounds are in a (solution, solutin) and act as if they have broken into individual pieces, the elements of the compound are called (electrolytes, electrolights).

8. The ability to record electrical charges is useful for (diegnostic, diagnostic) purposes.

F. Write the common symbol for the following elements.

1. sodium   _____   6. iron   _____

2. calcium   _____   7. iodine   _____

3. chlorine _____   8. phosphorous _____

4. hydrogen _____   9. potassium _____

5. oxygen   _____   10. carbon   _____

G. Answer the following questions about types of compounds.

1. The most important inorganic compound is _____.

2. List the four main groups of organic compounds.

_____

_____

_____

_____

3. The element always found in organic compounds is _____.

4. Explain the differences between a monosaccharide, disaccharide, and polysaccharide.

_____

_____

_____

_____

_____

_____

5. The form of glucose stored in the liver and muscle cells of the body is

   _____.

6. The sweetest of the simple sugars is _____.

7. An example of a polysaccharide found in plant tissue is _____.

8. The sugar found in DNA is _____, and the sugar found in RNA is

   _____.

9. A double sugar is formed from two simple sugars that lose a molecule of H_2O; this process is known as _____.

10. When a large molecule is broken down into smaller molecules by the addition of H_2O it is called _____.

H. Identify the compounds illustrated by the following symbols.

1. H_2SO_4 _____

2. NaCl _____

3. KOH _____

4. HCL _____

5. $C_{12}H_{22}O_{11}$ _____

6. CO_2 _____

7. NaOH _____

8. H_2O _____

9. $C_6H_{12}O_6$ _____

10. $NHCO_3$ _____

I. Compare the likenesses and differences between the following things.

1. Matter and energy

   _____

   _____

2. Acid and base

   _____

   _____

3. Element and compound

   _____

   _____

4. Ion and electrolyte

_____

_____

5. Protein and carbohydrate

_____

_____

6. Glucose and starch

_____

_____

7. CAT scan and MRI

_____

_____

8. DNA and RNA

_____

_____

J.   Carbohydrates are divided into three main groups: monosaccharides, disaccharides, and polysaccharides. Identify the group for each of the following sugars.

1. ribose _____		6. sucrose _____
2. cellulose _____		7. glycogen _____
3. maltose _____		8. lactose _____
4. fructose _____		9. dextrose _____
5. starch _____		

K.   Match the words in Column A with the most correct statement in Column B.

Column A	Column B
_____ 1. fats	a. consists of the elements C, H, O, and N
_____ 2. DNA	b. contains ribose sugar
_____ 3. phospholipid	c. triglycerides
_____ 4. protein	d. found in brain and nervous tissue
_____ 5. steroid	e. consists of the elements of C, H, O, N, and P
_____ 6. amino acid	f. genes for heredity
_____ 7. lysine	g. contains the elements C, H, and O
_____ 8. nucleic acid	h. essential amino acid
	i. the smallest molecule of protein
	j. contains cholesterol

L. Mark the following statements about acids, bases, and salts either true or false; correct any false statements.

_____ 1. An acid dissolved in water ionizes into positively charged hydronium ions or hydrogen ions and negatively charged ions of some other element.

_____ 2. Blue litmus paper does not change color in the presence of an acid.

_____ 3. A base is also called an alkali.

_____ 4. When dissolved in water, a base ionizes into negatively charged hydroxide ions and positively charged ions of a metal.

_____ 5. A base turns blue litmus paper red.

_____ 6. An acid and a base combine to form a salt and water; this reaction is called neutralization or exchange reaction.

_____ 7. In a neutralization reaction, hydrogen ions from the acid and hydroxide ions from the base join to form water.

_____ 8. In a neutralization reaction, the positive ions of the acid combine with the negative ions of the base to form a salt.

M. Complete the following chemical reactions and state whether each is an acid, base, or neutralization reaction.

1. $HCl + H_2O \rightarrow$ _____ $+ Cl^-$

   Reaction _____

2. $NaOH \rightarrow Na^+ +$ _____

   Reaction _____

3. Hydrochloric acid + _____ _____ $\rightarrow$ salt + water

   _____ + NaOH $\rightarrow$ _____ + _____

   Reaction _____

N. pH scale measures whether a solution is an acid or alkaline. Circle the correct answer.

1. Which pH is the most acidic?
   a. 5
   b. 7
   c. 9

2. Which pH is the most alkaline?
   a. 5
   b. 7
   c. 10

3. Water has a pH of:
   a. 7
   b. 7.3
   c. 6.9

4. Blood has a pH of:
    a. 7.0–7.1
    b. 7.35–7.45
    c. 6.9–7.0

5. A pH of 7 is considered:
    a. neutral
    b. acid
    c. base

O. Next to the following substances, state whether each is an acid or a base.

1. Milk _____

2. Baking soda _____

3. Gastric juice _____

4. Soap _____

5. Urine _____

6. Saliva _____

7. Vinegar _____

8. Carbonated beverages _____

9. Lemons _____

10. Milk of magnesia _____

P. Circle the key words related to the chemistry of living things.

```
o r g a n i c c a t a l y s t d a n
r b a s e c o m p o u n d r b i c e
g d y r t s i m e h c o i b e s e u
a m i n o a c i d f h g j k t a l t
n g m n o e l u c e l o m e a c e r
i e m y z n e l p y q u d s r c d a
c d n u c l e i c a c i d t d h i l
c i s p l u v e n e r g y w y a r i
o x t r x t r y m a t t e r h r a z
m o e o z i i a h b e z i n o i h a
p r r p d c d c f r e f f u b d c t
o d o e i m c o e n z y m e r e c i
u y i r o a j k m l i p i d a l a o
n h d t s n a b s a l t e f c a s n
d n a y u n i c e l l u l a r c o a
c d l e r f g h a l k a l i t s n c
l o r e t s e l o h c n i a j h o i
p h o s p h o l i p i d f k r p m d
```

Key Words

acid	lipid
alkali	matter
amino acid	molecule
atom	monosaccharide
base	multicellular
biochemistry	neutralization
buffer	nucleic acid
carbohydrate	organic catalyst
cholesterol	organic compound
coenzyme	pH scale
compound	phospholipid
disaccharide	polysaccharide
DNA	property
energy	RNA
enzyme	salt
fat	triglyceride
hydroxide	unicellular
ionize	

APPLYING THEORY TO PRACTICE

1. When we say an ion has a positive charge, what does this mean? The expression "opposites attract" occurs in chemistry. What does the expression mean when it applies to ions?

_____

_____

_____

_____

_____

2. As a society we worry about cholesterol, because we know it may clog the arteries and cause other health problems. Cholesterol has a function in our bodies. Name at least four functions of cholesterol. Explain why it is also considered a health risk.

_____

_____

_____

_____

3. You are employed in a group practice center. What nuclear medicine test would you expect to be ordered for the following conditions?
   a. Multiple sclerosis _____
   b. Epilepsy _____
   c. Visualization of the fetus _____
   d. Vascular blood flow _____
   e. Brain tumor _____

4. Explain the following tests.

Name of Test	Explanation	Special Instructions for the Patient
a. Sonography		
b. Positron emission tomography (PET)		
c. Computerized axial tomography (CAT)		
d. Magnetic resonance imaging (MRI)		

5. In which of the previous tests is an injection of a radionuclide given?

_____

6. Margaret is pregnant. At her obstetrics appointment, she reports a history of irregular menstrual cycles. To help determine her delivery date, the obstetrician will order what type of test?

_____

7. Diane is a young mother who brings her 7-year-old son to the pediatrician. She reports that he stares at the computer monitor and perhaps occasionally shakes. Diane reports that her son is addicted to video games. What type of diagnostic test will the doctor order for the child?

_____

8. John is a 70-year-old patient who has been complaining of abdominal pain. He has been in good health except for knee replacement surgery about a year ago. What must the doctor know about the knee replacement surgery before a nuclear imaging diagnostic test can be ordered?

_____

9. When babies are born today a cord sample of their blood is obtained. The mother is requested to take the blood home and keep it in the freezer compartment of the refrigerator. What is the purpose of this procedure?

_____

10. Ann has been trying to lose weight. Her problem is that she is addicted to sweets. What can she substitute for candy in a weight-reducing diet, to help satisfy her craving for sweets?

_____

SURF THE NET

Briefly summarize your findings from the suggested Web site or alternate sites. Follow the instructions at the suggested sites.

1. Understanding acids and bases may pose a problem. To help you understand this subject, go to
   http://astro.uchicago.edu/home/web/lenz/lesson.html

2. To obtain information on DNA basic structure and replication, go to
   http://www.eurekascience.com/

Lab Home Activities

1. Conduct a taste test at home for foods that contain acids or seem to be neutral. Invite another family member to join you in this experiment. Taste a piece of grapefruit, lemon, orange, strawberry, and banana.
   a. Which fruits seem to have an acid taste?
   b. Which fruits seem to be neutral?
   c. What taste are you experiencing?
   d. Is your family member having the same reaction?

2. Visually scan the food shelves at home. List at least 10 items that contain a type of carbohydrate. From the label, can you tell which type of carbohydrate it contains?

Cells

OVERVIEW

To study anatomy it is essential to understand the basic structure and function of the cell, the main parts of the cell and the organelles. It is important to understand how the cell obtains nutrients and reproduces through the process of mitosis.

Cells

The basic unit of structure and function of all living things is the cell. The cell has three major parts: cell membrane, nucleus, and cytoplasm.

Cell membrane is selective and semipermeable.

Nucleus is the control center of the cell; it has a nuclear membrane around it and contains the nucleoli and DNA.

Cytoplasm is a semifluid material between the cell membrane and the nucleus. Embedded in the cytoplasm are *organelles* that help a cell to function. The organelles include the *centrosomes, ribosomes, Golgi apparatus, endoplasmic reticulum, mitochondria, lysosomes, cytoskeleton,* and *peroxisomes.*

Functions of the Organelles

Centrosomes are active during mitosis.

Endoplasmic reticulum is a channel for transport of material in and out of the nucleus and cytoplasm.

Mitochondria supply energy for the cell in the form of ATP.

Golgi apparatus stores secretions for the cell.

Lysosomes digest protein molecules.

Ribosomes are the sites for protein synthesis.

Peroxisomes digest fats and detoxify harmful substances.

The *cytoskeleton* of microtubules and microfilaments is the internal framework.

Cell Division

There are two types of cell division. **Mitosis** is an orderly series of steps by which the DNA is precisely distributed to two new daughter cells, each with 46 chromosomes.

Meiosis is a special type of cell division of the germ cells, the ova and sperm. Each cell reduces to 23 chromosomes; when the ova and sperm unite there are 46 chromosomes.

Cell Movement

Movement of cell material through the semipermeable membrane occurs through passive and active processes. Passive processes that do not require energy are:

Diffusion: molecules move from an area of greater concentration to lesser concentration.

Osmosis: diffusion of water occurs across a semipermeable membrane from an area of higher concentration of a solution to an area of lower concentration of a solution.

Filtration: solutes and water move across a semipermeable membrane as a result of a mechanical force.

Active processes that require an energy source are:

Active transport: requires the energy of ATP to move molecules from an area of lower concentration to an area of higher concentration.

Phagocytosis: the cell engulfs particles; also known as *cell eating.*

Pinocytosis: the cell engulfs particles in solution; also known as *cell drinking.*

Effects of Aging

There are 30% fewer cells in the elderly.

Disorders of cell structure

Tumors are abnormal cell growths. They may be benign, confined to a local area, or malignant (cancer), when the cells move rapidly from one place to another.

ACTIVITIES

A.   Answer the questions or complete the statements regarding parts of the cell.

1. Name the three major parts of the cell.

   _____

   _____

   _____

2. The cell membrane is a double layer that regulates passage of molecules in and out of the cell; it is therefore called a _____ _____

   _____.

3. State the two major functions of the nucleus.

   _____

   _____

4. The nucleus contains _____ and protein.

5. The number of chromosomes in the nucleus is _____.

6. The outer layer of the nuclear membrane is continuous with the _____
   _____ of the cytoplasm.

7. Name the structure in the nucleus that contains the ribosomes.

   _____

8. Describe the cytoplasm.

   _____

   _____

9. The structures embedded in the cytoplasm that help cells function are the _____.

10. Do cells of the body have identical substances in their cytoplasm? Explain.

    _____

B. Organelles perform specific functions within the cell. Next to the following statements, write
the name of the organelle involved in that function from the list provided. A word may be used
more than once.

centrosome   lysosome
cytoskeleton   mitochondria
endoplasmic reticulum   peroxisomes
Golgi apparatus   ribosomes

1. Attached to the walls of the endoplasmic reticulum   _____

2. Detoxifies harmful substances   _____

3. The center for cellular digestion   _____

4. Forms internal framework   _____

5. Manufactures CHO and packages secretions   _____

6. Site for protein synthesis   _____

7. Transport of substances through the cytoplasm   _____

8. Site of cellular respiration and energy production   _____

9. Enzymes oxidize cell substances   _____

10. "Suicide bags"   _____

11. Role in cholesterol synthesis and fat metabolism   _____

12. Found in cells that need the most energy   _____

13. Abundant in gastric glands   _____

14. Plays an important role in mitosis   _____

C. Label and color the parts of the cell and the organelles. Use different colors for each part and organelle.

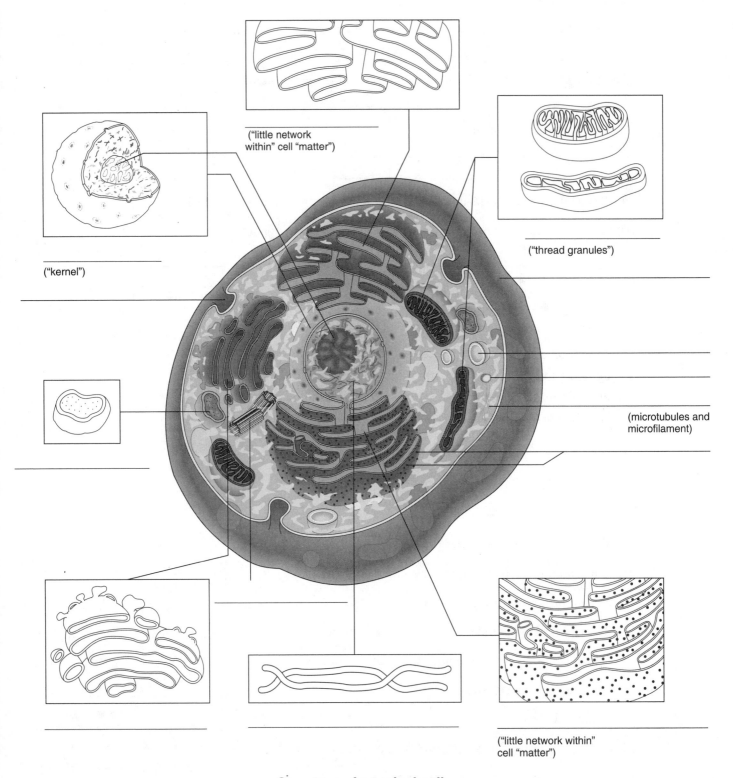

("little network within" cell "matter")

("kernel")

("thread granules")

(microtubules and microfilament)

("little network within" cell "matter")

Structure of a typical cell

D. Label the stage of mitosis and describe what is occurring in each stage.

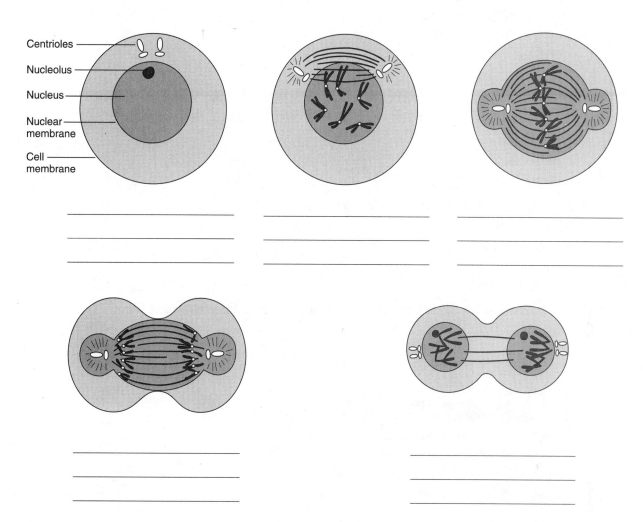

Centrioles

Nucleolus

Nucleus

Nuclear membrane

Cell membrane

_____   _____   _____

_____   _____   _____

_____   _____   _____

_____   _____

_____   _____

_____   _____

E. Circle the correct word in each of the following statements.

1. The process of cell division for somatic cells is called (mitosis, meiosis).

2. In the resting phase of cell division, an exact duplicate of each nuclear chromosome is made; this activity is called (replication, reproduction).

3. During prophase, two pairs of (centrioles, sentrioles) go to opposite ends of the cell.

4. In (telophase, metaphase), the chromosomes migrate to the opposite poles of the cell.

5. Cells produce proteins, such as albumin or globulin, that are essential to life through a process called protein (synthesis, synthisis).

F. Select the letter of the choice that best completes the statement.

1. The clear liquid fluid that fills the spaces around the chromatin and the nucleoli is:
   a. cytoplasm
   b. nucleoplasm
   c. nuclear membrane
   d. fatty substance

2. Water is essential for all cellular life, as water makes up:
   a. 50% to 70% of cytoplasm
   b. 60% to 70% of cytoplasm
   c. 70% to 80% of cytoplasm
   d. 70% to 90% of cytoplasm

3. In the nucleus of the cell, the DNA and protein are arranged in a loose state called:
   a. chromosomes
   b. chromatin
   c. centriole
   d. centrosome

4. An organelle with a smooth and rough side is the:
   a. mitochondria
   b. Golgi apparatus
   c. endoplasmic reticulum
   d. pinocytic vesicle

5. The two chromatids of each replicated chromosome are fully separated in the:
   a. telophase
   b. prophase
   c. anaphase
   d. interphase

6. All of the following types of cells undergo mitosis except:
   a. neurons of the nervous system
   b. goblet cells of the digestive system
   c. epithelial cells of the respiratory system
   d. epithelial cells of the reproductive system

7. The diffusion rate of molecules for a gas is:
   a. slower than liquids
   b. quicker than liquids
   c. slower than solids
   d. quicker than liquids and solids

8. Most intravenous fluids ordered by physicians are:
   a. hypertonic solutions
   b. isotonic solutions
   c. hypotonic solutions
   d. glucose and water solutions

9. The type of fluid ordered by the physician for a person with dehydration would be:
   a. hypertonic solution
   b. isotonic solution
   c. hypotonic solution
   d. glucose and water solution

10. The classification of drugs to treat cancers is known as:
    a. antineoplastics
    b. analgesics
    c. antibodies
    d. relaxants

G. Indicate whether the underlined word or phrase makes the statement true or false. If the statement is false, correct it.

_____ 1. Active transport that moves material across a cell membrane <u>does not require energy</u>.

_____ 2. An example of <u>diffusion</u> that moves molecules from an area of higher concentration to an area of lower concentration occurs when oxygen goes from the lungs to the bloodstream.

_____ 3. Osmosis is the diffusion of water through the cell membrane from an area of <u>higher</u> concentration of the solution to an area of lower concentration of the solution.

_____ 4. If a solution has the same number of sodium particles as the solute, the solution is said to be <u>hypertonic</u>.

_____ 5. In the process of <u>filtration</u>, the blood pressure forces the blood through the kidneys.

_____ 6. In the process of <u>phagocytosis</u>, the substances engulfed by the cell membrane are in solution.

_____ 7. Nerve cells are specialized to <u>respond</u> to stimuli.

_____ 8. Heart muscle cells <u>continue to divide</u> when they reach maturity.

_____ 9. A wart is a type of <u>benign</u> tumor.

_____ 10. A papilloma is a type of <u>malignant</u> tumor.

H. Match the activity with the word or phrase from the following list. An answer may be used more than once.

active transport   osmosis
diffusion   phagocytosis
filtration   pinocytosis

1. _____ The aroma of coffee percolating

2. _____ Blood passing through the kidney

3. _____ Cell drinking

4. _____ Exchange of oxygen from the blood to extracellular fluid

5. _____ Cell eating

6. _____ Putting sugar into a cup of tea

7. _____ Diffusion of water through a selective semipermeable membrane

8. _____ Process requires the energy of ATP

9. _____ Process by which white blood cells destroy bacteria

10. _____ Red blood cells placed in fresh seawater establish equilibrium

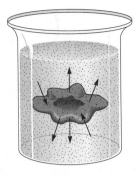

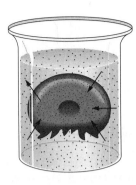

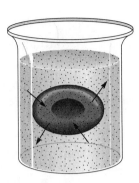

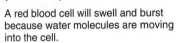
Water molecules

(seawater)

A red blood cell will shrink and wrinkle up because water molecules are moving out of the cell.

(freshwater)

A red blood cell will swell and burst because water molecules are moving into the cell.

(human blood serum)

A red blood cell remains unchanged, because the movement of water molecules into and out of the cell is the same.

I. Read the description below the illustration of the red blood cell in plasma. State the type of solution illustrated.

J. Answer the following questions.

1. Describe what occurs in a hypertonic solution.

   _____

   _____

2. Describe what occurs in a hypotonic solution.

   _____

   _____

3. Describe what occurs in an isotonic solution.

   _____

   _____

K. Fill in the blanks with the appropriate word.

Active transport is a way in which cells may obtain nutrients and excrete their waste products. In this process, molecules move across the cell membrane from an area of _____ concentration to _____ concentration, which requires _____ in the form of the compound _____.

Think of the cell membrane as a bridge. A molecule from _____ the cell wants to cross over the bridge and get _____ the cell. To do this, the molecule needs an escort called a _____ molecule. Arm in arm they go across the cell membrane; once inside the cell the escort _____ the molecule at the _____ surface of the membrane. The escort then returns to the other side of the bridge to wait for the next molecule that wants to cross the bridge or cell membrane.

L.   Match the term in Column A with the word or phrase from Column B.

Column A	Column B
_____ 1. cytoskeleton	a. contains DNA and protein
_____ 2. nucleolus	b. structure to help cells function
_____ 3. ATP	c. enzyme that detoxifies harmful substance
_____ 4. metaphase	d. needed for active transport
_____ 5. peroxisome	e. a strain of replicated chromosome
_____ 6. cancer	f. malignant cells that move rapidly
_____ 7. chromatid	g. the nuclear membrane disappears
_____ 8. nucleus	h. malignant cells
_____ 9. metastases	i. contains ribosomes
_____ 10. organelles	j. internal framework of the cell

M.   Complete the story on the cell using the following list of words.

cell	lysosomes
cell membrane	mitochondria
centriole	nucleus
cytoplasm	organelles
cytoskeleton	peroxisomes
DNA	phagocytosis
endoplasmic reticulum	ribosomes
Golgi apparatus	RNA

THE C.E.L.L.

The employment agency sent Ms. Glucose to a new plant that was hiring temporary help for the season. When Ms. Glucose arrived at the C.E.L.L. Plant Company, she noticed that the entryway had a most peculiar door. It appeared to have little holes throughout and a sign posted saying, "Do not push anything through this _____."

As a huge gap appeared on the side of the entryway and engulfed her, she heard a voice say, "Do not worry about that; it is only _____ up to his old tricks." Ms. Glucose was finally inside this strange company; the air was very humid and all the surfaces felt slippery. A receptionist, Mr. RNA, appeared and said the atmosphere was especially suited for the kind of work done at the C.E.L.L. Company; this substance is called _____.

The receptionist said, "Stick with me; I am called Mr. _____, and I will take you on a tour of the plant." They hopped aboard a tramlike car labeled E.R.T., which meant _____ _____ _____. Along the way Ms. Glucose was introduced to the various departments.

Mr. RNA said, "We are like chipmakers; we manufacture peppy little proteins that are then changed into many other products." The first stop was a place where they synthesized the protein; it was called _____ department. As they traveled, Ms. Glucose noticed scaffolding throughout. She was told it was _____, which forms the internal framework of the plant.

In one area the air was hot and full of energy. The head of the department was dressed like a super hero in keeping with the _____ or powerhouse division of the plant. In quick order they went to the packing plant or _____ _____ division, which uses carbohydrate packing material to send packages from the factory.

Before a product is shipped, it passes through two quality-control rooms. One is the _____ room, which bathes the product in oxidase material; this helps to remove harmful impurities. The other is the _____ room, which checks to see whether additional cellular digestion is required for the final product.

The final destination was a special walled room in the center, called the president's office. It was guarded by two identical-looking secretaries called Ms. and Mr. _____ . The president's office is also known as the _____ of the plant. The president of the company is known as _____ , because he dictates what happens in that factory. Ms. Glucose thanked Mr. RNA for the tour, but she really did not think she was ready for a job at C.E.L.L., the home of the _____ .

APPLYING THEORY TO PRACTICE

1. In the classroom Rebecca dropped her purse and her bottle of nail polish fell out and broke. The smell of nail polish soon permeated through the classroom. This is an example of the process of _____ .

2. When preparing coffee, the coffee is placed into a lined basket in a holder, very hot water is poured over the coffee, and the liquid and some of the solids pass through to the serving container. This is an example of the process of _____ .

3. Courtney has an infection in her right ear. Her white blood cells will help control the infection by eating up the harmful bacteria. This process is known as _____ .

4. Much discussion has developed since the arrival of a sheep named Dolly. The procedure that made Dolly started with genetic material from the nucleus of a sheep's udder cell which was fused with an egg (nucleus removed) to create the embryo which became Dolly. This process is known as _____ .

5. Anthony had a biopsy done on a mole removed from his left shoulder. The doctor reports that the mole is the size of a quarter, it is localized, there was no lymph node involvement, and it had not metastasized. The doctor was using the classification system known as

_____ .

6. Lucille has been diagnosed with leukemia. The doctor's will use her stem cells as therapy to treat her particular type of leukemia. The type of stem cells found in adults is known as _____ stem cells.

7. Our body cells do not all reproduce at the same rate. How frequently do our intestinal, skin, muscle, and nerve cells reproduce?

_____

_____

_____

8. The doctor has just told your aunt that she has a neoplasm and that it must be biopsied. If the biopsy is positive, the doctor has told her that she may need surgery and other treatment.

   a. Define a neoplasm.

   _____

   _____

   _____

   b. Describe the types of neoplasm.

   _____

   _____

   _____

   c. What is the implication of a positive biopsy?

   _____

   _____

   _____

   d. List some of the early signs of cancer.

   _____

   _____

   _____

   e. Name the tests used to diagnose cancer.

   _____

   _____

   _____

   f. Discuss some of the treatment modalities for cancer.

   _____

   _____

   _____

   g. List some of the major problems involved with cancer treatment.

   _____

   _____

   _____

9. What is the purpose of the United States Genome Project?

   _____

   _____

   _____

10. Societal concern is arising from new genetic research. Answer the following questions regarding this issue.

   a. Who should have access to personal genetic information?

   b. Who owns and controls genetic information?

   c. How does personal genetic information affect an individual's and society's perception of that individual?

QUOTE FALLS CREATION

Solve the puzzle by using the letters in the column to unscramble the quotation.

Movement of materials across cell membranes

T	A	A	C		O					H	W			S	M		E		
T	A	L	T	T	U	N	N		O	N	L	D	I	F	F	R	O	N	C	N	N
M	R	R	E	I	O	L	F	T	I	I	O	V	E	R	R	C	C	I	N	A	E
N	O	R	E	A	I	O	E	S	H	M	G	O	E	E	F	U	O	O	O	C	N

SURF THE NET

Briefly summarize your findings from the suggested Web sites, or choose alternate sites for the following topics.

1. To help you understand cell knowledge, go to http://www.members.tripod.com/~detonn/cell.htm

2. For a microscopic appearance of cancer cells, go to http://www.newscenter.cancer.gov/sciencebehind/cancer/cancer19.htm

3. For information about stem cell research, go to http://www.webmd.lycos.com/content/article and search for articles on the subject.

Tissues and Membranes

OVERVIEW

Tissues are groups of cells similar in shape, size, structure, intercellular material, and function. Two layers of tissue form membranes. A group of organs act together to form an organ system.

Tissues are groups of cells that are similar in shape, size, structure, intercellular material, and function. Four main types of tissue are as follows:

Epithelial tissue protects the body by covering internal and external surfaces. Covering and lining types include *squamous, cuboidal,* and *columnar;* glandular or secretory types include *exocrine* and *endocrine* glands.

Connective tissue includes cells whose intercellular material (matrix) supports and connects organs. Types include adipose areolar, dense fibrous, supportive (bone and cartilage), and vascular (blood and lymph).

Muscular tissue provides movement and produces body heat.

Nervous tissue reacts to stimuli and conducts messages.

Membranes are formed by two layers of tissues. Types of membranes are *epithelial,* which produce either mucous or serous secretions, *cutaneous,* and *connective.*

Mucous membranes are also called mucosa, and include respiratory mucosa, gastric mucosa, and intestinal mucosa.

Serous membranes are the pleural (lining thoracic cavity), pericardial (lining heart cavity), and peritoneal (lining abdominal cavity).

Cutaneous membranes are related to skin.

Connective membranes are made of two layers of connective tissue. Synovial membrane is one type; it lines the joint cavities.

Human Organism

The formation of the human organism progresses from different layers of complexity: from atom to molecule to organelle to cell to tissue to organ to organ system to human organism. Organs are several tissues grouped together to perform a single function.

Organ Systems

Organ systems are groups of organs that act together to perform specific related functions. The following are types of organ systems.

Skeletal: serves as the framework; forms blood components and stores minerals.

Muscular: provides for movement and produces body heat.

Digestive: prepares food for absorption by the body through mechanical and chemical means.

Respiratory: takes in oxygen and gives up carbon dioxide.

Circulatory: carries oxygen and nutrients to the cell and carries waste away from the cells.

Reproductive: reproduces organisms.

Excretory: eliminates the waste products of metabolism.

Endocrine: manufactures hormones to regulate body activity.

Nervous: communicates, coordinates, and controls body activities through response to stimuli.

Integumentary: protects the body and is a sensory organ.

Degree of Tissue Repair

The degree of tissue repair depends on the damage or injury and where it is located. Types of repair include the following:

Primary repair takes place in a clean wound; a scab will form if a larger area of tissue is involved. Damage to deeper tissues requires the edges of the wound to be brought together with sutures.

Secondary repair is required in deeper and larger wounds; healing takes place by the process of granulation.

Vitamins necessary for tissue repair include A, B, C, D, E, and K.

ACTIVITIES

A.   Answer the following questions regarding tissues.

1. Cells, when grouped according to their structure, intercellular material, and function, are called _____.

2. Name the four major types of tissue and their primary functions.

    _____

    _____

    _____

    _____

3. Circle the mismatched pairs.

   Squamous/outer layer of skin
   Cuboidal/lining of digestive tract
   Columnar/part of the respiratory tract
   Glandular/secrete hormones
   Exocrine/thyroid gland
   Endocrine/adrenal gland

B. Each diagram illustrates the structure of the tissue. Label the diagram with the name of epithelial tissue and its function in the body.

1. Cube-shaped cells.

   Name of tissue: _____

   Function:_____

   _____

   _____

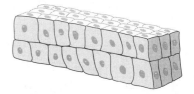

2. Elongated with the nucleus generally near the bottom; often ciliated.

   Name of tissue: _____

   Function:_____

   _____

   _____

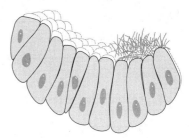

3. Flat, irregularly shaped cells

   Name of tissue: _____

   Function:_____

   _____

   _____

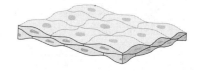

4. Glandular tissue specialized to secrete hormones.

   Name of tissue: _____

   Function:_____

   _____

   _____

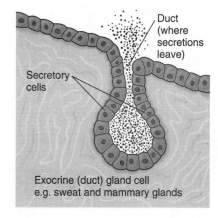

Duct (where secretions leave)

Secretory cells

Exocrine (duct) gland cell
e.g. sweat and mammary glands

C. In the glandular type of epithelial tissue there are two types of glands that secrete. Write EX next to exocrine glands and EN next to endocrine glands.

_____ mammary gland

_____ thyroid gland

_____ sweat gland

_____ salivary gland

_____ adrenal gland

D. Connective tissue ranges from loose, ordinary type to that which can bear weight. Write one or two sentences describing each type of connective tissue and where it is located in the body.

1. Adipose tissue

    Description: _____

    _____

    _____

    _____

    Location: _____

    _____

    _____

Cytoplasm
Collagen fibers
Nucleus
Vacuole (for fat storage)

2. Areolar (loose connective) tissue

    Description: _____

    _____

    _____

    _____

    Location: _____

    _____

    _____

Mast cell
Reticular fibers
Collagen fibers
Fibroblast cell
Plasma cell
Elastic fiber
Matrix
Macrophage cell

3. Dense fibrous tissue

    Description: _____

    _____

    _____

    _____

    Location: _____

    _____

    _____

Closely packed collagen fibers

Fibroblast cell

4. Supportive—bone tissue

Description: _____

_____

_____

_____

Location: _____

_____

_____

Bone cell
Cytoplasm
Nucleus
Bone lacunae

5. Supportive—cartilage tissue
   a. Hyaline

Description: _____

_____

_____

_____

Location: _____

_____

_____

Cells (chondrocytes)
Matrix
Lacuna (space enclosing cells)

   b. Fibrocartilage

Description: _____

_____

_____

_____

Location: _____

_____

_____

Chondrocytes
Dense white fibers

   c. Elastic cartilage

Description: _____

_____

_____

_____

Location: _____

_____

_____

Elastic fibers
Chondrocyte
Nucleus

6. Vascular tissue

a. Blood

Description: _____

_____

_____

_____

Location: _____

_____

_____

Erythrocytes   Thrombocytes   Lymphocyte
                (platelets)

Neutrophil   Monocyte   Basophil

Eosinophil

b. Lymph

Description: _____

_____

_____

_____

Location: _____

_____

_____

Red blood cells
White blood cell
Blood
capillary   Lymph

Cells

Lymph
capillary

E. Match the description in Column A with the type of tissue in Column B.

Column A	Column B
_____ 1. blood	a. adipose tissue
_____ 2. fibroblast	b. fasciae
_____ 3. elastic, single fibers	c. ligaments
_____ 4. tissue sheet that wraps around muscle bundles	d. bone tissue
_____ 5. flexible, white fibrous protein	e. collagen
_____ 6. holds bones together at joints	f. simple squamous tissue
_____ 7. connects muscle to bone	g. vascular tissue
_____ 8. calcified by mineral salts	h. areolar tissue
_____ 9. fat	i. tendon
_____ 10. lymphocytes and granulocytes	j. elastin
	k. columnar epithelial tissue
	l. lymph tissue

F. Complete the following statements in reference to muscle tissue.

1. Cardiac muscle tissue is _____ and involuntary; it makes up the
    _____ of the heart.

2. _____ muscle tissue is nonstriated and _____ .

3. Skeletal muscle tissue is _____ and _____ .

G. Nervous tissue has two unique characteristics. Describe them.

_____

_____

_____

H. Circle the correctly spelled word in each of the following statements about membranes.

1. (Epithelial, Epethelial) membranes are classified as mucous or serous depending on their secretion.

2. The mucous membranes line (surfuses, surfaces) and spaces that lead to the outside of the body.

3. The type of secretion of the mucous membrane is mucus, which (lubicates, lubricates) and
    protects the lining, especially of the (respiratory, risporatory) tract.

4. The portion of serous membrane that covers the organs is called (viseral, visceral) lining, and
    the portion that lines the cavity is called (parietal, parital).

5. Lining the thoracic cavity is the (plural, pleural) membrane.

6. The (precardial, pericardial) lining is in the heart cavity.

7. The lining of the abdominal cavity is the (peritoneal, peratoneal) membrane.

8. The connective membrane lining the joint cavity is (sinovial, synovial).

I. Label the following diagram. Color the serous membranes blue and the mucous membranes red.

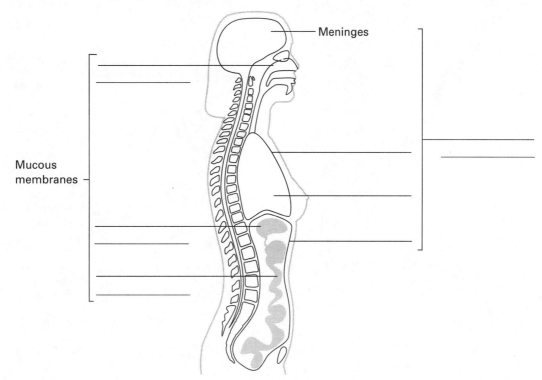

J. Label the diagram from the simple to the complex in the development of the organism.

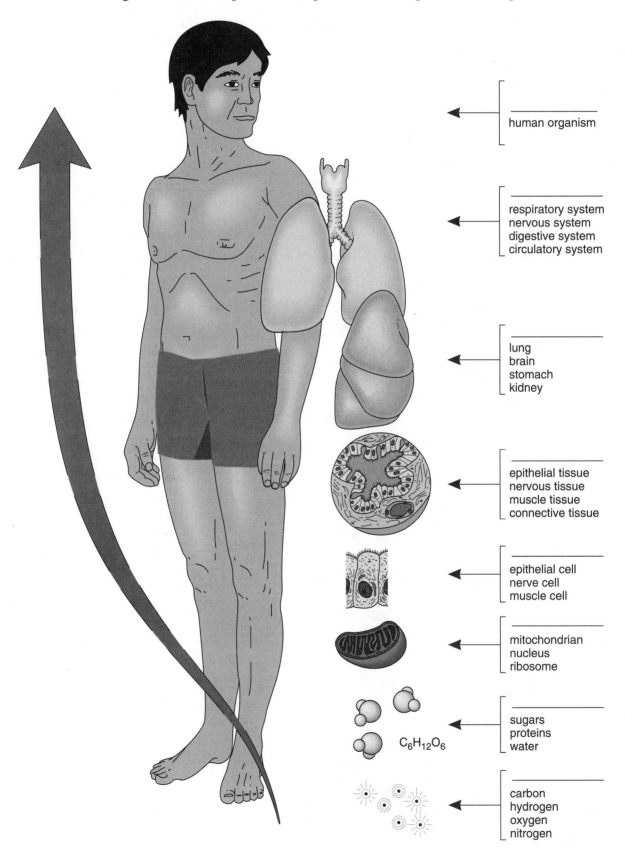

_____
human organism

_____
respiratory system
nervous system
digestive system
circulatory system

_____
lung
brain
stomach
kidney

_____
epithelial tissue
nervous tissue
muscle tissue
connective tissue

_____
epithelial cell
nerve cell
muscle cell

_____
mitochondrian
nucleus
ribosome

_____
sugars
proteins
water

$C_6H_{12}O_6$

_____
carbon
hydrogen
oxygen
nitrogen

K. Complete the following table on the body systems.

The Ten Body Systems

SYSTEM	SYSTEM FUNCTIONS	ORGANS
Skeletal	_____ _____ _____	Skull, spinal column, ribs and sternum, shoulder girdle, upper and lower extremities, pelvic girdle
_____	Determines posture; produces body heat; provides for movement.	_____ _____ _____
Digestive	_____ _____ _____	Mouth (salivary glands, teeth, tongue), pharynx, esophagus, stomach, intestines, liver, gallbladder, pancreas
Respiratory	_____	_____ _____
Circulatory	_____ _____	Heart, arteries, veins, capillaries, lymphatic vessels, lymph nodes, spleen
_____	Removes waste products of metabolism from body.	_____ _____
Nervous	_____ _____	Brain, nerves, spinal cord, ganglia
_____	Manufactures hormones to regulate organ activity.	_____ _____ _____
Reproductive	Reproduces human beings.	*Male* *Female* ____ ____ ____ ____ ____ ____ ____ ____ ____ ____ ____ ____ ____ ____
Integumentary	_____ _____ _____ _____ _____	Epidermis, dermis, sweat glands, oil glands

L. Select the letter of the choice that best completes the statement.
  1. The following tissue does not repair itself but is replaced with scar tissue:
    a. muscle
    b. bone
    c. heart
    d. nervous

2. The type of tissue involved in a simple skin injury is:
   a. columnar epithelial
   b. cuboidal epithelial
   c. ciliated columnar epithelial
   d. squamous epithelial

3. In primary repair of deeper tissues, fibroblast cells help make new collagen fibers within:
   a. 24–48 hours
   b. 48–72 hours
   c. 72–96 hours
   d. 96–120 hours

4. In secondary repair, an open wound with large tissue loss heals by:
   a. the granulation process
   b. stratified squamous epithelial cells dividing
   c. capillary fluid drying and sealing the wound
   d. edges of the wound being sewn together

5. A bactericidal action helps to reduce the risk of infection by:
   a. reducing the number of bacteria
   b. destroying bacteria
   c. keeping the area clean
   d. increasing blood supply to the area

M. Specify which vitamins (A, B, C, D, E, or K) help in each healing process.

_____ 1. This vitamin is necessary for healing bones because it enhances calcium absorption from food.

_____ 2. This vitamin is important for the normal production of collagen and repair of connective tissue.

_____ 3. This vitamin is helpful in the replacement of epithelial tissues, for example, in the lining of the respiratory tract.

_____ 4. Thiamine, nicotinic acid, and riboflavin are vitamins of this group and generally promote the well-being of the individual.

_____ 5. This vitamin aids in blood clotting and helps to prevent excessive blood loss.

_____ 6. This vitamin promotes healing by its action as an antioxidant protector.

APPLYING THEORY TO PRACTICE

1. Name the type of tissue:
   a. on the end of your nose   _____
   b. in the lining of your mouth   _____
   c. on your skin   _____
   d. on the lobe of your ear   _____
   e. on your fingers   _____

2. A mother brings her son into the emergency room with a deep, clean cut. She asks how this wound is ever going to heal. Explain to the mother the process of primary repair for deeper tissue.

   _____

   _____

   _____

   _____

3. Bridgette has been vomiting for 10 hours. Her father brings her to the emergency room where she is diagnosed with gastritis. The tissue involved in the inflammation of the stomach is _____

4. Mrs. Givia, age 85, resides in a Skilled Nursing Faculty. She complains of being cold even though the temperature in the room is 76°F. Mrs. Givia may have lost some of her subcutaneous fat, which is part of _____ tissue.

5. Victoria has been exercising and lifting weights. Her right shoulder develops pain and stiffness. The doctor states she has bursitis of the shoulder joint. The membrane lining the shoulder joint is called _____.

SURF THE NET

Briefly summarize your findings at these Web sites and explore other Web sites for information in these areas.

1. For a review of cells, tissues, and membranes, go to
   http://www.Training.seek.cancer.gov/module_anatomy/unit2_1_cell_functions.html

2. For a tissue quiz, go to http://www.science.nhmccd.edu/biol/dropdrag/quizl.htm

3. To review body systems, search the Web for sites that provide additional information on the topic. Bookmark your favorites for reference in later chapters.

Integumentary System

OVERVIEW

The skin is our protective covering and is called the integumentary system. It is tough, pliable and multi-functional.

Functions of the Integumentary System

Functions of the integumentary system include the following:

Covering and protecting tissue from infection and dehydration

Regulating body temperature

Helping to manufacture vitamin D

Acting as a site for nerve receptors

Acting as a site for temporary storage of fat, glucose, water, and salts

Screening out harmful rays of sunlight

Absorbing certain drugs and other chemicals

Structure of the Skin

Skin consists of two major divisions: the epidermis and the dermis. The *epidermis,* or epithelial tissue, is the outermost layer of skin. It is avascular and contains keratin and melanocytes. The *dermis* is connective tissue containing collagen, elastic fibers, nerve endings, hair follicles, and oil and sweat glands. The *subcutaneous* or hypodermal layer is not a true part of integumentary, but is made of loose connective and adipose tissue.

Appendages of the Skin

Characteristics of the skin include appendages such as hair, nails, and certain glands. *Hair* consists of the hair root, shaft, and three layers. *Nails* are keratinized plates that cover the ends of the fingers and toes. *Sweat glands,* or sudoriferous glands, help to cool skin through perspiration. *Sebaceous glands* secrete sebum, which lubricates the skin and hair.

Effects of Aging

The sebaceous glands secrete less sebum skin becomes fragile and dry. Loss of subcutaneous fat results in lines and wrinkles. The vascular network decreases in response to heat and cold.

Skin Disorders

Skin can be host to numerous disorders, including those that follow:

>*Acne vulgaris*—oversecretion of the sebaceous glands; mostly seen in adolescents
>*Athlete's foot*—contagious fungal infection, usually found between the toes
>*Dermatitis*—inflammation of the skin
>*Eczema*—noncontagious, inflammatory skin disease
>*Impetigo*—acute, inflammatory, and contagious skin disease mostly seen in babies and young children
>*Psoriasis*—chronic inflammatory disease
>*Ringworm*—contagious fungal infection with circular patches
>*Urticaria* or *hives*—skin reaction of itchy wheals, usually the response to an allergen
>*Boils*—bacterial infection of a hair follicle
>*Shingles* (*herpes zoster*)—skin eruption due to a viral infection of the nerve endings
>*Herpes*—viral infection seen as a fever blister or cold sore
>*Genital herpes*—viral infection of the genital area

Skin Cancer

Skin cancers are the most common combined cancer in the United States. They include the following types.

>*Basal cell*—most common and least malignant
>*Squamous cell*—arises from the epidermis, grows rapidly
>*Melanoma*—malignant, occurs in the pigmented cells of the skin; may appear as a brown or black irregular patch

>All are associated with overexposure to ultraviolet light.

Burns

Burns result from radiation, heat, chemicals, or electricity. First degree burns involve the epidermis; redness, swelling, and pain are present. Second degree burns may involve the epidermis and dermis; pain, redness, swelling, and blistering are present. Third degree burns involve complete destruction of the skin; they are life threatening because of fluid loss and infection.

Skin Lesions

Different types of skin lesions include bulla, macule, nodule, papule, pustule, ulcer, tumor, vesicle, and wheal.

ACTIVITIES

A. Answer the following questions regarding skin functions.

1. List the seven functions of the skin.

_____

_____

_____

_____

_____

_____

_____

2. Which functions provide protection for the body?

_____

3. How does the skin regulate body temperature?

_____

_____

B. Match the letter from Column B that best completes the statement in Column A.

Column A	Column B

One square centimeter of skin contains:

_____ 1. nerve endings to record pain   a. 3,000
_____ 2. sensory apparatuses for heat   b. 4
_____ 3. sensory cells at the end of nerve fibers   c. 25
_____ 4. yards of nerves   d. 200
_____ 5. pressure apparatuses   e. 12

C. Complete the following statements about skin layers.

1. The stratum corneum is replaced by a nonliving substance that forms a waterproof covering. It is called _____.

2. The stratum corneum destroys bacteria because it is slightly _____.

3. Thickening of the outer layer of skin in a concentrated area is called a _____; if the thickening grows inward it is called a _____.

4. The stratum germinativum is thrown into ridges known as _____. This characteristic can be used for _____.

5. The muscle attached to the hair follicle is known as the _____ _____ muscle.

6. Another name for the dermis layer is _____.

7. Sudoriferous glands are exocrine glands that produce _____. Their ducts extend to form _____ on the skin.

8. The average amount of sweat produced per day is _____ ml.

9. The hypodermis layer contains fat and is also called the _____ layer.

10. Sebaceous glands produce _____, which lubricates the skin, keeping it _____ and _____.

D. Label the diagram of the skin and color its parts.

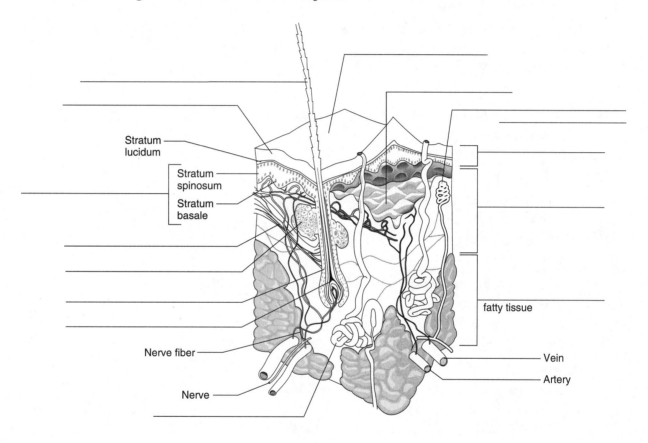

E. Next to each structure, state whether it is part of the hair or nails.

1. Cuticle layer or cortex _____

2. Hard, keratinized plate _____

3. Shaft in dermis _____

4. Medulla or inner layer _____

5. Elongated epidermal cell _____

F.   Select the letter of the choice that best completes the statement.

1. The body's first line of defense is formed by the:
    a. stratum germinativum
    b. stratum corneum
    c. stratum spinosum

2. Light-skinned people generally have a greater proportion of:
    a. keratin in the skin
    b. pheomelanin in the skin
    c. eumelanin in the skin

3. The hair is composed of three layers:
    a. cuticle, cortex, and medulla
    b. keratin, cuticle, and cortex
    c. cuticle, cortex, and dermis

4. The name given to glands found in the ear canal is:
    a. sebaceous
    b. mammary
    c. ceruminous

5. The epidermal layer of melanocytes, keratinocytes, and Langerhans cells is:
    a. stratum granulosum
    b. stratum spinosum
    c. stratum lucidum

6. The best way to prevent the spread of infection is by handwashing for:
    a. 15–20 seconds
    b. 15–25 seconds
    c. 15–30 seconds

7. Underarm odor is caused by the interaction of:
    a. bacteria and secretion from sudoriferous glands
    b. bacteria and secretion from hair follicles
    c. bacteria and secretion from ceruminous glands

8. Impetigo is a contagious condition and is caused by:
    a. fungus or yeast infection
    b. viral infection
    c. staphylococcus or streptococcus organism

9. Burns that involve only the first layer of skin are:
    a. first degree
    b. second degree
    c. third degree

10. A painful condition that occurs around the nerve endings is:
    a. herpes simplex
    b. shingles
    c. psoriasis

G. Circle the correctly spelled word in each of the following statements.

1. Sweat glands are also called (sudoriferous, suderferous) glands.

2. (Athete's foot, Athlete's foot) is a contagious fungal (infection, enfection) characterized by the formation of small (blesters, blisters) between the fingers and toes.

3. A (chronic, cronic) noncontagious (inflammatory, inflamatory) skin disease is called (eczema, ekzema). In this condition, the skin becomes dry, itchy, and (scaly, scaley).

4. (Psoriasis, Psorasis) is a skin disease in which there are red patches covered by (silvery, silverey) white scales.

5. A person may develop (urticaria, uticaria) or hives as the result of an (allergic, alergic) reaction.

H. Next to each description write the correct disorder.

acne vulgaris	dermatitis	impetigo
boils or carbuncles	eczema	psoriasis
cherry angiomas	genital herpes	ringworm
decubitus	herpes	shingles

1. This nonspecific rash could be caused by chemicals such as soap or by stress.

   _____

2. This disorder of the sebaceous gland plugs the opening of the gland and occurs primarily during adolescence. _____

3. The treatment for this condition, which has raised, circular patches with crusts, is griseofulvin. _____

4. As one ages these benign red bumps may appear on the skin. _____

5. This bacterial infection of a hair follicle or sebaceous gland becomes deeply embedded in the skin. _____

6. The onset of this chronic inflammatory condition affects mainly the elbows and knees, and may be triggered by stress or trauma. _____

7. This chronic noncontagious inflammation of the skin is often caused by sunlight.

   _____

8. This skin condition accompanied by severe pain is known as herpetic neuralgia.

   _____

9. These blistered areas result from lying in the same position without shifting weight.

   _____

10. This inflammatory contagious skin condition seen in babies is characterized by the appearance of vesicles that rupture and develop distinct yellow crusts. _____

I. Mark the following statements as either true or false; correct the false statements.

_____ 1. The most common type of cancer is skin cancer.

_____ 2. Basal cell carcinoma usually has a recovery rate of 75%.

_____ 3. Squamous cell cancer is usually found on the face.

_____ 4. Malignant melanoma is a tumor that may appear as a brown or black irregular patch.

_____ 5. Squamous cell cancer rarely metastasizes.

_____ 6. The usual treatment for skin cancer is surgical removal and radiation.

J. The following illustrations show types of burns. Match them with the letter of the accompanying skin diagram.

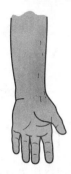

First degree, superficial

_____

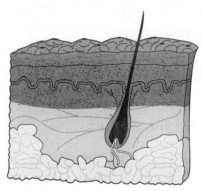

A. Blistered, skin moist, pink or red

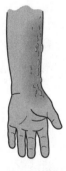

Second degree, partial thickness

_____

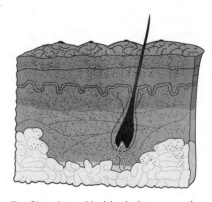

B. Charring, skin black, brown, red

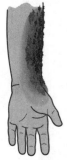

Third degree, full thickness

_____

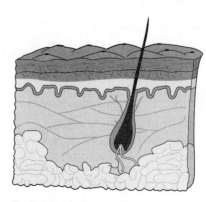

C. Skin red, dry

K. Match the words in Column A with the most correct statement in Column B.

Column A	Column B
_____ 1. ringworm	a. solid, abnormal mass of cells
_____ 2. papule	b. loss of skin surface may extend to the dermis
_____ 3. wheal	c. fluid-filled raised area
_____ 4. pustule	d. raised, itchy, circular patches with crusts
_____ 5. macule	e. brown or black irregular patch
_____ 6. vesicle	f. flat spot, flush with skin area, that is a different color
_____ 7. melanoma	g. elevated solid area
_____ 8. psoriasis	h. discrete pus-filled area
_____ 9. ulcer	i. reddish patches with silvery scales
_____ 10. tumor	j. itchy, temporarily elevated area

L. State whether the treatment or statement is for first, second, or third degree burns.

_____ 1. Life-threatening situation

_____ 2. Pain medication and dry, sterile dressing

_____ 3. Application of cold water

_____ 4. Prevention of contracture and fluid replacement

_____ 5. Healing generally in 2 weeks

_____ 6. Eschar present

_____ 7. Redness, swelling, and blistering

M. Label and describe the following skin lesions.

1. _____

_____

_____

_____

Example: Lipoma, erythema, cyst

2. _____

_____

_____

_____

Example: Stage 2 pressure ulcer

3. _____

_____

_____

_____

Example: Insect bite or a hive

4. _____

_____

_____

_____

Example: Freckle

5. _____

_____

_____

_____

Example: Carcinoma (such as advanced breast carcinoma); **not** basal cell or squamous cell of the skin

6. _____

_____

_____

_____

Example: Herpes simplex, herpes zoster, chickenpox

7. _____

_____

_____

_____

Example: Acne, impetigo, furuncles, carbuncles, folliculitis

8. _____

_____

_____

_____

Example: Contact dermatitis, large second degree burns, bulbous impetigo, pemphigus

9. _____

_____

_____

_____

Example: Warts, elevated nevi

N. Use the words from the following list to complete the rhyme about functions of the skin.

bacteria   hot
bones   protective
difference   receptors
elastic   sunburn
evaporation   vitamin D
harmful   wrinkled

Think about your skin and what comes to mind?
How does your _____ coat stand the test of time?

From baby's skin, smooth, _____, and smelling so sweet
to aging skin, _____, dry, and not feeling too neat.

It helps protect us from the _____ rays of the sun
but your skin thinks a _____ is definitely not fun.

The skin helps us manufacture _____ for free
and that keeps our _____ strong and healthy.

When our bodies are _____, it cools us by perspiration,
a process completed by _____.

The sense _____ present let us know
the _____ between a soft touch or a hard blow.

All this time you never thought too much about your skin.
It keeps us well by preventing _____ from getting in.

APPLYING THEORY TO PRACTICE

1. A factor in the color of a person's skin is determined by its pigmentation. Explain the mechanism of skin pigmentation and the factors that affect it.

_____

_____

_____

_____

2. A friend obtains a nicotine patch to help her stop smoking. She asks you how something she puts on her skin can work. How do you reply?

_____

_____

_____

_____

3. Skin disorders are visible for all to see. Parents whose children have eczema worry about what others will think when they see patches on the skin. What could you do to relieve a parent's stress?

   _____

   _____

   _____

   _____

4. A father brings his son to the emergency center with first, second, and third degree burns. Name the major complications that result from second and third degree burns. Discuss the treatment for and complications of second and third degree burns. When a person has third degree burns, he or she is not in pain; explain the reason.

   _____

   _____

   _____

   _____

5. Bryan, age 15, visits the school nurse because of his cysts and pimples. What condition does Bryan have and what is the cause? Is there a treatment for this condition? _____

   _____

6. Rebecca will soon be 14 years old. For her birthday she wants a gift certificate to a tanning salon. Her father says no. He explains to Rebecca that prolonged exposure to this activity may lead to what condition? _____ _____

7. Jodi is a 35-year-old mother who comes to the doctor's office because of a rash on her forearms and hands. She has been using a new type of dishwashing soap. What is the doctor's diagnosis of Jodi's condition? _____ _____

8. Your 90-year-old grandmother has had a stroke and has been in a nursing home for about 3 months. On your last visit you noticed a red, blistered area on the back of her leg. Name your grandmother's skin condition, its stage of development, and the proper treatment.

   _____ _____

9. Aliya is 3 years old and attends preschool. Her mother notices several bumps on her arms that contain watery fluid. This condition may be a skin disease often seen in infants and young children. Name the condition. Will Aliya be able to attend preschool with this condition?

   _____

   _____

   _____

10. Frank, age 75, complains of pain, which seems to be in his chest and back. Frank also has small blistered areas on his chest. What is the family doctor's diagnosis of Frank's condition?

    _____

SURF THE NET

Briefly summarize your findings from these suggested Web sites, or choose alternate sites for the following topics.

1. To better understand skin anatomy, go to
   http://www.gen.umn.edu/faculty_staff/jensen/1135/webanatomy/wa_cell_chem/
   wa_web_skin1.htm

2. For more information on pressure ulcers go to
   http://www.expertpages.com/news/decubitus_ulcer.htm

3. For burn classification information, go to
   http://www.cooltheburn.com/learn/about/classify.html

4. To take a burn awareness quiz, go to http://www.burnresource.com/quiz.html

Skeletal System

OVERVIEW

The **skeletal system** is the bony framework within the body. It is composed of 206 bones.

Functions of the Skeletal System

Functions of the skeletal system are as follows:

    Supporting body structures
    Protecting internal organs
    Serving as an attachment for muscles
    Storing minerals, calcium, and phosphorous
    Acting as a hemopoiesis site of blood cell formation
    Aiding movement

Bone Formation

Bone is made of organic and inorganic material.

Structure of a Long Bone

Long bone consists of the following:

    Diaphysis is the hollow, cylindrical shaft of a long bone.
    Epiphysis is at each end of the diaphysis; it contains the red marrow.
    Medullary canal is the center of the shaft, and has yellow marrow. The lining is called the *endosteum.*
    Compact bone is hard bone surrounding the medullary canal.
    Spongy bone is that which remains when some of the hard bone dissolves.
    Periosteum is fibrous tissue covering the outside of the bone.

Growth

Long bone grows from the diaphysis to the epiphysis. Bone cells include the following:

> *Osteoblasts* are bone cells that deposit new bone.
>
> *Osteoclasts* are bone cells that secrete enzymes that split the bone minerals into calcium and phosphorous.
>
> *Osteocytes* are bone cells that help to maintain bone as a living tissue.

Bone Types

Long, flat, irregular, and short are types of bones.

Parts of the Skeleton

Axial. The axial skeleton includes skull, vertebral column, sternum, ribs, and hyoid.

The *skull* is divided into cranial and facial bones.

> The cranium has 8 bones in the frontal, parietal, temporal, occipital, ethmoid, and sphenoid areas.
>
> The face has 14 bones in the nasal, maxilla, mandible, lacrimal, zygomatic, and palatine areas.

The *vertebral column* includes cervical (7), thoracic (12), lumbar (5), sacrum (1), and coccyx (1) bones.

The *sternum* includes the breastbone (1).

The *ribs* include true ribs (7), false ribs (3), and floating ribs (2).

The *hyoid* is a U-shaped bone (1) in the neck.

Appendicular. The appendicular skeleton includes shoulder girdles, arms, wrists, hands, pelvic girdle, legs, ankles, and feet.

The *shoulder girdle* includes the clavicle (2) and scapula (2).

The *arm* includes the humerus (2), a bone in the upper arm; the radius (2), which runs up the thumb side of the forearm; the ulna (2), a larger bone of the forearm.

The *hand* has carpals (16), 8 small bones that make up each wrist; metacarpals (10), each hand has 5, which make up the palm; phalanges (28), each hand has 14, which make up the fingers.

The *pelvic girdle* (1) is made up of ilium, ischium, and pubis bones.

The *upper leg* is the femur or thigh bone, the longest and strongest bone in the body.

The *lower leg* has the tibia, or shin bone, and fibula, the smaller bone of the lower leg.

The *ankle* has tarsals (14), each ankle having 7 tarsals; the calcaneus is the heel bone.

The *foot* has metatarsals (10), each foot having 5 bones arranged to make up the arch; and phalanges (28), each foot having 14, which make up the toes.

LIGAMENTS AND TENDONS

Ligaments connect bones and cartilage; tendons connect muscles to bones.

Joints and Related Structures

A **joint** is the point of contact or articulation between two bones. Related structures of joints are as follows:

Articular cartilage is the smooth slippery cap of cartilage that covers the two joint surfaces.

Articular capsule is the fibrous connective tissue that encloses the two joint surfaces; it is lined with synovial membrane.

Ligaments are fibrous bands that connect bones and cartilage.

Tendons are fibrous cords that connect muscle to bone.

Types of Joints

Types of joints include diarthroses, amphiarthroses, and synarthroses.

Diarthroses are freely movable joints. Types of diarthroses are ball and socket, which have the greatest degree of freedom (hip); hinge, which moves in one direction (elbow, knee); pivot, which has an extension rotating in a second arch-shaped bone (axis); and gliding, in which flat surfaces glide across each other (vertebrae).

Amphiarthroses are partially movable joints (symphysis pubis).

Synarthroses are immovable joints; they connect bone by fibrous connective tissue (sutures of the skull).

Types of Joint Movement

Following are the various types of joint movement.

Flexion decreases the angle between two bones.

Extension increases the angle between two bones.

Abduction is movement away from the midline.

Adduction is movement toward the midline.

Circumduction includes flexion, extension, abduction, and adduction.

Rotation moves bones around a central axis.

Pronation is the palm downward or backward.

Supination is the palm forward or upward.

Effects of Aging

After the age of 40, bone mass and density begin to shift, which leads to osteoporosis and a change in posture. Joints also become less mobile and flexible.

Disorders of the Bones and Joints

Fractures. A **fracture** is a break in the bone. Types of fractures include greenstick, simple, compound, or comminuted.

Bone and Joint Injuries. Bone and joint injuries include the following:

Dislocation. Bone is displaced from its proper position in a joint.
Sprain. Ligaments are torn from their attachment to the bone.
Strain. A minute tear occurs in muscle.

Bone Diseases. The body can be afflicted with various bone diseases.

Arthritis is an inflammatory condition of one or more joints. Types include *rheumatoid,* a chronic autoimmune disease, and *osteoarthritis,* articular cartilage degeneration.
Gout occurs due to uric acid crystals deposited in a joint cavity; the most commonly affected site is the great toe.
Rickets is when bones are soft due to lack of vitamin D.
Slipped disk is a cartilage disk that ruptures or protrudes out of place and puts pressure on a spinal nerve.
Whiplash is trauma to the cervical vertebrae.
Abnormal curvatures of the spine include *kyphosis,* a humped curvature in the thoracic area of the spine; *lordosis,* an exaggerated inward curvature in the lumbar region of the spine; and *scoliosis,* a lateral curvature of the spine.
Osteoporosis is loss of calcium and phosphorous in the bone causing brittleness.
Osteomyelitis is inflammation of the bone.
Osteosarcoma is cancer of the bone.

ACTIVITIES

A. List the five functions of the skeletal system.

_____

_____

_____

_____

_____

B. Mark the following statements as either true or false. Correct any false statements.

_____   1. The cranium protects the brain, the outer ear, and parts of the eye.

_____   2. Bones act as passively operated levers to move the body.

_____ 3. Once a bone such as your humerus is formed, the bone tissue is never replaced unless the bone is broken.

_____ 4. Red marrow, which manufactures blood cells, is found in irregular bones, the sternum, and hip bones.

_____ 5. Some of the mineral salts found in bone are calcium, sodium, and phosphorous.

c. Using the following words, numbers, and abbreviations, complete the story on bone growth and development.

Ca	cartilage	epiphysis	ossification	25%
Na	center	fontanel	osteoblast	35%
Mg	collagen	growth	osteoclast	65%
Fe	diaphysis	lateral	white blood cells	8
Zn	enzyme	marrow cavity	yellow	
P	epiphyseal plate			

I AM A FEMUR

From the time of my beginning, my part was made of fibrous material called collagen, which is secreted by _____. Four weeks into my embryonic life, _____ was deposited between my fibers. Into my jellylike self, about the _____ th week, mineral salts began to creep; I felt myself getting harder. I have heard that this process is called _____. The mineral salts belonged to a family called elements; they went by the special names of _____, _____, _____, and _____. My makeup is _____% organic material and _____% inorganic material, mineral salts, and water.

I started to grow from the _____ of my shaft toward my end, which go by the name _____. I continue to grow along a special plate called the _____ zone. I would look funny just growing toward the ends, so I started to grow around the middle, too. The osteoblast added bone to the outer surface of my middle, which has a special name like my end; it is called _____. Then something starts eating me up inside like acid indigestion. I have _____ spitting out their little _____, causing a hole in my middle, called the _____ _____. This cavity gets filled with _____ marrow, and _____ _____ _____ come to live in it.

D. Label the long bone diagram and match the letter that corresponds to the description.

_____ 1. Lining of the marrow cavity

_____ 2. Located in the center of the shaft

_____ 3. Shaft

_____ 4. Site of manufacture of blood cells

_____ 5. Articular layer covering epiphysis

_____ 6. Ends of long bone

_____ 7. Hard bone dissolves, leaving this type

_____ 8. Tough fibrous covering of bone

_____ 9. Fat storage center

_____ 10. Bone surrounding the medullary canal

C _____

D _____

E _____

F _____

Artery _____

G _____

H _____

I _____

J _____

A _____

B _____

E. Complete the statements with the correct word or words.

1. One function of the skeletal system is to store minerals such as calcium; this helps maintain the blood _____ _____.

2. The process of blood cell formation in the bones is called _____.

3. The organic substance of bone gives it a degree of _____.

4. A hard blow to the cranium may cause a _____.

5. Blood vessels that nourish the osteocytes or bone cells travel to the area through the

_____ _____.

6. The wrist and ankle are cubelike in shape; they also may be classified as _____ bones.

7. Irregular bands of connective tissue that hold the bones in place during infancy are called

_____.

8. The bone that forms part of the nasal septum is called the _____.

9. On the _____ or second cervical vertebrae is the _____ process, which permits us to nod our heads.

10. On the lower cartilaginous part of the breastbone or _____ is the _____ process, an important landmark in CPR.

F.　Answer the following questions about the skeleton.

1. Label the bones of the skeleton. Color the bones of the axial skeleton blue and the appendicular skeleton yellow.

2. How many bones are in the skeleton? _____

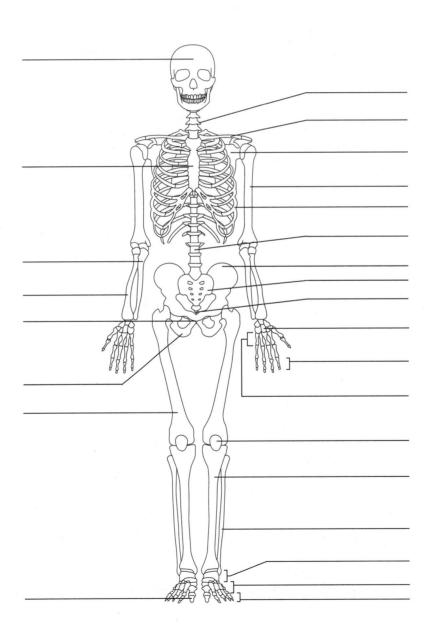

G.   Label and color the bones of the skull. Color the bones of the cranium blue and the bones of the face yellow.

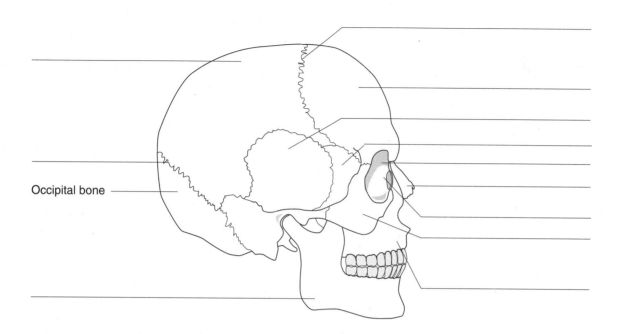

Occipital bone

H.   Using the diagram of the cranial bones, match the name of the bone with the following information. Also indicate the quantity of each structure.

1.   The dome shape of all of these bones protects this. _____

2.   This bone forms part of the nasal septum. _____   # _____

3.   Organs of hearing are protected by this bone. _____   # _____

4.   Forms the roof and sides of the cranium. _____   # _____

5.   Protector of the anterior portion of the brain, the forehead. _____   # _____

6.   It has the foramen magnum, the opening through which the spinal cord connects with the brain. _____   # _____

7.   All the bones of the cranium connect with it. _____   # _____

I.   The face has two palatine bones, which form the roof of the mouth with the maxilla. The hyoid bone is a U-shaped bone in the posterior portion of the mouth. Write the name of the other bones of the face in the statements that follow. Include the number of bones involved.

1.   The cheek bones also form the lateral walls of the orbit of the eye. _____   # _____

2.   These bones hold the ducts from which our tears fall. _____   # _____

3.   The upper jaw, which also forms the hard palate. _____   # _____

4.   These bones make up the side walls of the nasal cavity. _____   # _____

5. These bones join to form the bridge of the nose. _____ # _____

6. Lower jaw; the only movable bone in the face. _____ # _____

7. Forms part of the nasal septum. _____ # _____

J. Label the bones of the vertebrae. Color the cervical vertebrae red, the thoracic vertebrae green, the lumbar vertebrae blue, the sacrum yellow, and the coccyx orange.

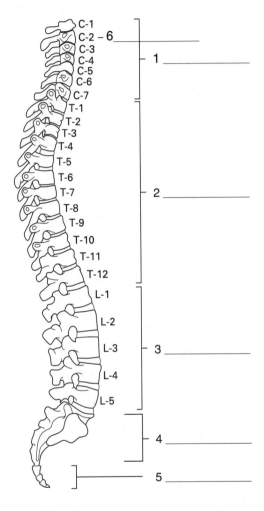

K. Label a typical vertebra: **body, foramen,** and **transverse process.**

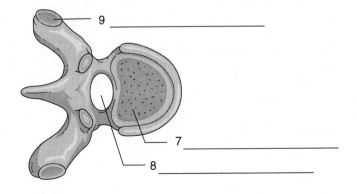

L.   Using the labels from the previous two diagrams, match the correct number with the statement.

	Number
1. Large solid part of the vertebrae	_____
2. Second cervical vertebra	_____
3. Forms posterior portion of the pelvic girdle	_____
4. Central opening in a vertebra	_____
5. Tailbone	_____
6. Above foramen, two winglike projections	_____
7. Articulate with the ribs	_____
8. Have large and heavy bodies	_____
9. First seven vertebra	_____

M.   Label the rib cage and sternum in the following diagram. Color the true ribs blue, the sternum green, the false ribs gold, the costal cartilage gray, and the floating ribs brown. Why do the ribs have names like true, false, and floating? _____

_____

_____

N.   Answer the following questions regarding the appendicular skeleton.

1. The two bones that form the shoulder girdle are the _____ or

_____ _____ and the _____

or _____ _____. Feel these bones on yourself. The

location where they meet serves as the attachment point for the arms.

2. Label the following diagrams of the arm and hand. List the bones of the upper extremity from distal to proximal. Indicate how many of each there are in one upper extremity.

a. phalanges   # _____   d. _____   # _____

b. _____   # _____   e. _____   # _____

c. _____   # _____   f. _____   # _____

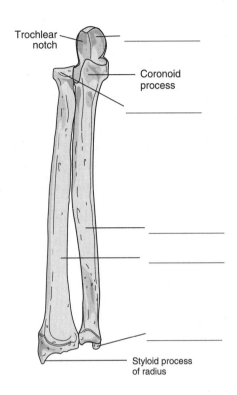

Trochlear notch

Coronoid process

Styloid process of radius

Anterior view

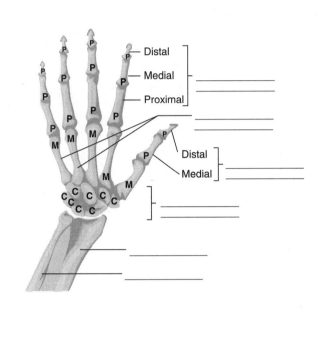

Distal

Medial

Proximal

Distal

Medial

Bones of the left hand

O. Label the diagrams of the bones and structures of the pelvic girdle.

1. Name the bones that fuse together to form the innominate or hip bone. _____

_____

2. The hip bone joins with what axial bone to form the pelvic girdle? _____

3. Name the part on the pelvic girdle where the head of the femur fits in to form a ball-/-and-socket joint. _____

False pelvis

Inlet of true pelvis

Wider angle
in female

FEMALE

P. Refer to the skeleton in Figure 6–3 in your textbook. Name the bones of the lower extremity from proximal to distal.

1. femur

2. _____

3. _____

4. _____

5. _____

6. _____

7. _____

Q. Answer the following questions regarding bones of the feet.

1. Look at the bones of your foot. Take a few steps. What structure is responsible for giving spring to your step? Is this structure also in the palms of your hand?

   _____

   _____

2. Label the diagram of the foot bones. Color the tarsals red, the metatarsals yellow, and the phalanges blue. Coloring the phalanges blue indicates what condition may be coming?

   _____

   _____

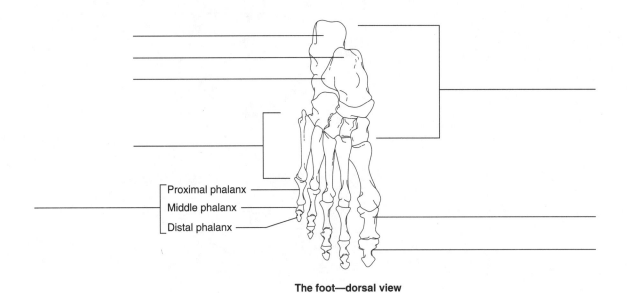

Proximal phalanx ─────
Middle phalanx ─────
Distal phalanx ─────

The foot—dorsal view

R. Match the terms in Column B with the statements in Column A regarding joint structure, tendons, and ligaments.

Column A	Column B
_____ 1. movable joint	a. amphiarthrosis
_____ 2. immovable joint	b. synovial membrane
_____ 3. fibrous band that binds joints	c. disk
_____ 4. partially movable joint	d. tendon
_____ 5. lining the articular cartilage	e. diarthrosis
_____ 6. example of pivot joint	f. suture of the skull
_____ 7. fibrous cord connects muscle to bone	g. ligament
_____ 8. elastic material between vertebrae	h. radius and ulna

S. In the following diagram, label the joint movement illustrated and match the letter to the correct statement.

_____ 1. Allows a bone to move around one central axis

_____ 2. Act of increasing the angle of two bones

_____ 3. Movement toward the midline

_____ 4. Act of bringing two bones closer together

_____ 5. Movement away from the midline

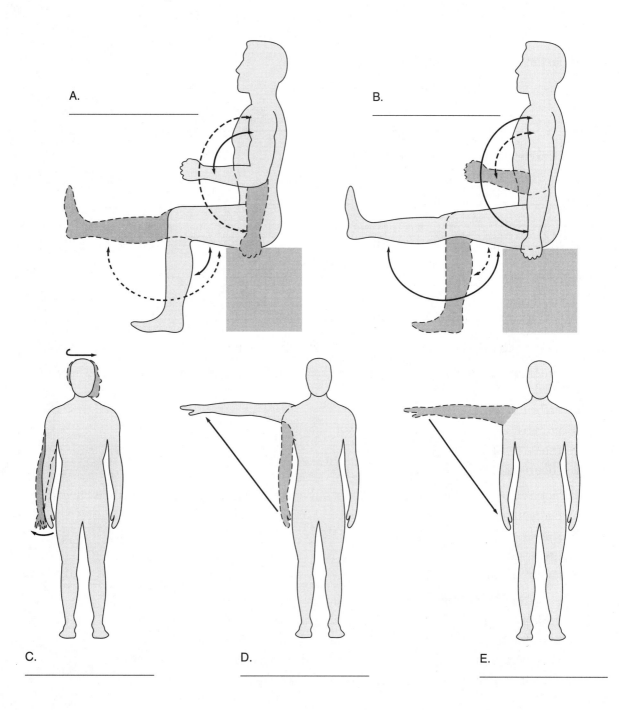

T. Compare the differences between each of the following:

1. Male pelvis and female pelvis

   _____

   _____

   _____

2. Ball-and-socket joint and hinge joint

   _____

   _____

   _____

3. Synarthrosis joint and amphiarthrosis joint

   _____

   _____

   _____

4. Axial skeleton and appendicular skeleton

   _____

   _____

   _____

5. Kyphosis and lordosis

   _____

   _____

   _____

U. Select the letter of the choice that best completes the statement.

1. An inflammation of the clefts in the connective tissue between muscle, tendons, and ligaments is called:
   a. arthritis
   b. bursitis
   c. osteoarthritis
   d. rheumatoid arthritis

2. A fracture in which the bone is partly bent but never penetrates through the skin is called:
   a. compound
   b. simple
   c. greenstick
   d. comminuted

3. The treatment for a fracture may be closed reduction, which is:
   a. bony fragments brought into alignment by manipulation
   b. bony fragments brought into alignment by surgical intervention
   c. bony fragments brought into alignment by devices such as wires or screws
   d. bony fragments brought into alignment by a pulling force

4. A chronic autoimmune disease that affects the joints is:
    a. bursitis
    b. tendinitis
    c. osteoarthritis
    d. rheumatoid arthritis

5. An exaggerated inward curvature of the spine is:
    a. scoliosis
    b. lordosis
    c. hunchback
    d. kyphosis

6. In osteoporosis the mineral density of the bone is reduced; the average woman by age 55 has lost:
    a. about 20% of her bone mass
    b. about 25% of her bone mass
    c. about 30% of her bone mass
    d. about 35% of her bone mass

7. Rickets, a disease in which bones become soft, is caused by lack of:
    a. vitamin A
    b. vitamin B
    c. vitamin C
    d. vitamin D

8. A traumatic injury to the cervical vertebrae is:
    a. whiplash
    b. gout
    c. kyphosis
    d. herniated lumbar disc

9. An infection of the bone is called:
    a. gout
    b. arthritis
    c. osteosarcoma
    d. osteomyelitis

10. An injury to the joint in which the ligaments are torn from the attachments to the bone is called a:
    a. dislocation
    b. sprain
    c. strain
    d. fracture

V.   Complete this two-part puzzle.

1. In Column B, write the correct name of the bone or bones from the descriptions in Column A.

2. Use the words from Column B for the word search. When you are finished, the remaining letters in the word search will give you a message.

Word Search

```
M E T A C A R P A L S S
U O A M E L E H B O I N
I E I S M U L A S O V F
H T B U H B C L E T L S
C A I I P I I A H A E U
S L T D P F V N U R P E
I E N A D I A G M S A N
C U L R A R L E E A T A
S A L U P A C S R L E C
K N E L E T A L U S L L
T L O F E M U R S N L A
P U B I S S L A P R A C
```

Column A	Column B
wrist bones	_____
fingers	_____
collarbone	_____
shoulder bone	_____
rotates around ulna	_____
kneecap	_____
heel bone	_____
pelvic girdle (3 bones)	_____
	_____
	_____
palms of the hand	_____
small lower leg bone	_____
broad tarsal bone	_____
bone with olecranon process	_____
articulates with scapula	_____
longest, strongest bone	_____
ankle bones	_____
shin bone	_____
structure is different in males and females	_____

APPLYING THEORY TO PRACTICE

1. A person fell off a ladder and broke one-third of the bones of the appendicular skeleton. How many bones would be broken?_____

2. When you think about the skeletal system, bones come to mind. Yet there are two other body systems affected by the skeletal system. Name them and their connection to the skeletal system.

_____

_____

_____

3. The patient comes to the doctor's office with a condition known as athlete's foot. If one-fourth of the toes of both feet show this condition, how many toes are involved?

_____

4. Anthony, age 4, is brought to the emergency room. He fell off his bike, and a piece of bone has broken through the skin of his lower arm. The doctor states that it is what type of fracture? Explain an open reduction to the parents.

   _____

   _____

   _____

   _____

5. As people age, they are often affected by some form of arthritis. At a health fair you are asked to do a presentation of the following. Briefly describe each.
   a. Arthritis and the different types of arthritis

   _____

   _____

   _____

   Symptoms:

   _____

   _____

   Treatment:

   _____

   _____

   b. Arthroscopy

   _____

   c. Arthroplasty

   _____

   _____

6. Employment studies indicate that there will be great career opportunities for physical therapists in the future. What are the duties of a physical therapist? Are there any obstacles to this career path?

   _____

   _____

   _____

7. Leslie, age 50, suffers from chronic low back pain. A friend suggests she try acupuncture. Leslie is afraid of having needles put into her back. Explain to Leslie how acupuncture may alleviate her pain.

   _____

   _____

   _____

8. While driving home from work, Nora had to brake suddenly to avoid hitting the car in front of her. Nora's neck immediately began to hurt. What type of injury did Nora sustain? Explain what happens to the skeletal structures in this type of injury.

   _____

   _____

9. Steven, age 45, has difficulty in putting on his left shoe, because his big toe is swollen and painful. After a visit to the doctor, Steven is diagnosed with gout. Explain to Steven the cause and treatment of gout.

   _____

   _____

   _____

10. Pat is contemplating arthroscopic surgery for a problem she is having with her left knee. She knows you are a registered nurse and asks if you know anything about this procedure and if it is beneficial. How do you respond to Pat?

   _____

   _____

   _____

SURF THE NET

Briefly summarize your findings from these web sites, or choose alternate sites for the following topics.

1. For additional facts about the skeletal system, go to
   http://www.gen.umn.edu/faculty_staff/jensen/1135/webanatomy/wa_skeleton

2. For signs and symptoms and other information about concussions go to
   http://www.edc.gov/ncipe/tbi/default.htm

3. For updates on arthritic devices, go to http://www.raacademy.com?use_assistive_devices

4. For scoliosis signs and treatment, go to http://www.spineuniverse.com

Muscular System

OVERVIEW

Muscles comprise nearly half of our body weight and are responsible for all movement.

Functions of the Muscular System

Functions of the muscular system include:

Being responsible for all body movement
Giving the body form and shape
Producing most of the body heat

Types of Muscle

Muscle is one of three types:

Skeletal is striped or striated, multinucleated, attached to the bones of the skeleton, and voluntary.
Smooth (visceral) is nonstriated, has one nucleus, and is involuntary.
Cardiac is striated and branched, found only in the heart, and is involuntary.

Characteristics of muscle are contractibility, extensibility, elasticity, and irritability. Muscles only pull, they never push.

Attachment and Function of Skeletal Muscle

Origin is the part of the muscle that is attached to a fixed structure, moving the least during a muscle contraction. *Insertion* means it is attached to the movable part of the bone, moving the most during a muscle contraction.

Muscle Pairs

Muscles are arranged in pairs.

Prime mover creates movement in a single direction / *antagonist* creates movement in the opposite direction (biceps and triceps).

Flexor flexes or bends a joint / *extensor* extends or straightens a joint.

Levator raises a body part / *depressor* lowers a body part.

Contraction of Skeletal Muscle

The sources of energy for muscle contractions are glucose, oxygen, and ATP. Movement occurs as a result of myoneural stimulation and contraction of muscle proteins.

Muscle Fatigue

Muscle fatigue is caused by an accumulation of lactic acid, a waste product of muscle metabolism.

Muscle Tone

Muscles are always in a state of slight contraction and ready to pull. The following terms describe muscle tone.

Isotonic contraction: muscles shorten and contract.

Isometric contraction: tension increases; muscle does not shorten.

Atrophy: muscles shrink from disuse.

Hypertrophy: muscle fibers increase in size from overuse.

Naming of Skeletal Muscles

Muscles are named by location, size, direction of fibers, number of origins, location of origin and insertion, and action.

Muscles of the Head and Neck

Examples of muscles of the head and neck include the following:

Frontalis controls facial expressions.

Masseter controls mastication.

Sternocleidomastoid moves the head.

Muscles of the Upper Extremities

Examples of muscles of the upper extremities include the following:

Deltoid moves the shoulder.

Biceps moves the arm.

Flexor carpi moves the wrist, hand, and fingers.

Muscles of the Trunk

Examples of muscles of the trunk include the following:

Diaphragm helps in breathing.

Rectus abdominus compresses the abdominal cavity.

Muscles of the Lower Extremity

Examples of muscles of the lower extremity include the following:

Gluteus maximus moves the upper leg.

Sartorius moves the lower leg.

Tibialis anterior moves the ankle.

Peroneus longus moves the ankle, foot, and toes.

See tables in text book for a more complete listing of muscles.

Exercise and Therapy

Exercise of muscles will improve strength and efficiency of muscles and circulation. *Massage therapy* may provide health benefits as well as offering a form of physiotherapy.

Intramuscular Injections

Intramuscular injections may be given in the following sites: deltoid, gluteus medius, and vastus lateralis.

Effects of Aging

Over time, the muscle system experiences a gradual decrease in the number of muscle fibers, which results in a loss of strength and energy.

MusculoSkeletal Disorders

Rehabilitation or therapeutic exercise will help damaged or injured muscles. Following are various types of musculoskeletal disorders.

Muscle strain is a tear in the muscle.

Muscle spasm is a sustained contraction of the muscle.

Myalgia is used to describe muscle pain. Fibromyalgia is a collection of symptoms, the most definite of which is chronic muscle pain lasting 3 or more months.

Hernia is an organ protrusion through a weak muscle wall. Types are abdominal, hiatal, and inguinal.

Flat feet (talipes) is a weakening of the leg muscles that support the arch of the foot.

Tetanus (lockjaw) is an infectious disease characterized by continuous spasms of voluntary muscles.

Torticollis (wry neck) is an inflammation of the trapezius and/or sternocleidomastoid muscles.

Muscular dystrophy is a group of diseases in which the muscle cells deteriorate.

Myasthenia gravis is progressive muscular weakness and paralysis.

Recreation Injuries.   *Tennis elbow (lateral epicondylitis)* is inflammation of the tendon that connects the arm muscle to the elbow.

Shin splints is injury to the muscle tendon in front of the tibia.

Rotator cuff disease is inflammation of the group of tendons that surround the shoulder joint.

ACTIVITIES

A.   Label the diagrams of the muscle tissue. List three structural features of each type of muscle tissue and location in the body where each type is found.

1. Name of tissue: _____

   _____

   Features: _____

   _____

   _____

   _____

   Location: _____

   _____

2. Name of tissue: _____

   _____

   Features: _____

   _____

   _____

   _____

   Location: _____

   _____

3. Name of tissue: _____

   _____

   Features: _____

   _____

   _____

   _____

   Location: _____

   _____

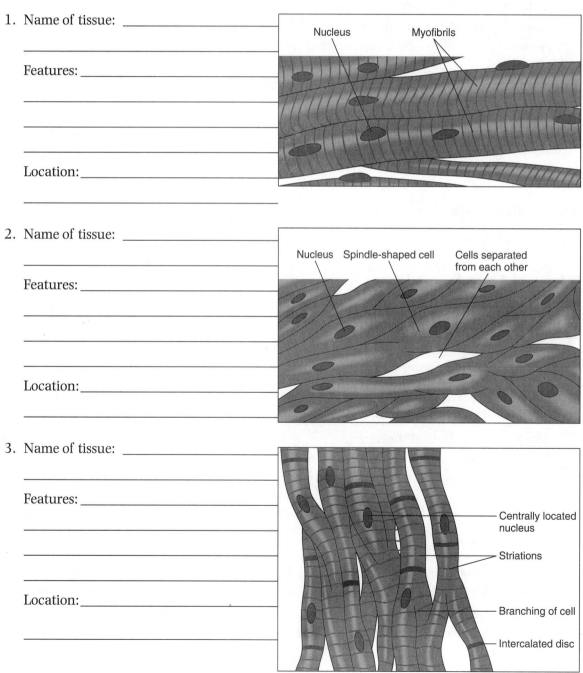

B. Name the four common characteristics of the muscle cells.

_____

_____

_____

_____

C. Place the correct word or words next to the following statements; make a selection from the list provided.

antagonist	elasticity	insertion	smooth muscle
cardiac muscle	excitability	origin	synergist
contractibility	extensibility	prime mover	tendons
dilator	fasciae	skeletal muscle	

1. A characteristic shared with nerve cells; the ability to respond to a stimulus.

_____

2. This structure contains membranes fused at places called intercalated disks; a communication system at the fused area will not permit the cells to act independently. _____

3. The ability of a muscle to return to its original length after stretching. _____

4. The ability of muscles to be stretched. _____

5. Muscles only pull and never push; they are attached to the bones of the skeleton by nonelastic cords. _____

6. The part of the muscle attached to a fixed point on the bones; the least movable part during a contraction. _____

7. The ability of this muscle to cause the diameter of blood vessels to decrease on contraction.

_____

8. Muscles that open and close to control the passage of substances. _____

9. The ability of the muscle to shorten, which reduces the distance between the parts of its contents. _____

10. The part of the muscle attached to the movable part of the bone; it is the most movable during a contraction. _____

D. Using the following words, complete the story about steps in muscle contraction. Words may be used more than once.

action potential	fatigue	motor	positive
adenosine triphosphate	glucose	neurotransmitter	sarcolemma
ATP	lactic acid	original	sodium
contraction	length	pain	synaptic cleft
cramps			

For muscles to work, they need a stimulus from a _____ nerve and a source of energy that is _____ _____, also known as _____. The muscle cell also requires oxygen and _____.

Between the nerve cell's fiber, the axon, and the muscle cell is a neuromuscular junction called the _____ _____. When the nerve impulse reaches the end of the axon, it releases a chemical called _____. This chemical diffuses across the junction and attaches to the cell membrane, the _____. This action makes the membrane temporarily permeable to _____. The muscle cell now has excessive _____ ions, which upsets the electrical condition; the cell now has an _____ _____.

Skeletal muscle contraction begins with the action potential that travels along the _____ of the muscle fiber, from one end of the cell to the other. This energy source results in the _____ of the muscle cells.

When the action potential is ended, the muscle cell relaxes and returns to its _____ length.

Lactic acid is a product of muscle contractions that is changed back to _____ and other substances with the help of oxygen. Sometimes when there is too much muscle activity and not enough of an oxygen supply (anaerobic), a buildup of _____ _____ will occur in the blood. This condition results in muscle _____ and _____. A person needs to stop, rest, and take in enough oxygen to complete the catabolism of lactic acid and relieve the muscle _____.

E. Make the following statements about muscle tone accurate by circling the correct word.

1. Muscles are (always, sometimes, never) in a state of partial contraction.

2. In an isometric contraction, the tension in a muscle (decreases, increases, stays the same). The muscle (does, does not) shorten.

3. In an isotonic muscle contraction, the muscle (does, does not) shorten.

4. When muscles are flaccid, they are (weak, strong).

5. In atrophy, the muscle (increases, decreases) in size from disuse.

6. In hypertrophy, the size of the muscle (shrinks, enlarges). The number of cells is (the same, more, less) as a result of over exercising.

F. Muscles are named by location, size, number of origins, location of origins and insertions, and action. Match the muscles in Column A with the clues given in Column B.

Column A	Column B
_____ 1. frontalis	a. action
_____ 2. gluteus maximus	b. direction of fibers
_____ 3. triceps brachii	c. raises the body
_____ 4. sternocleidomastoid	d. location
_____ 5. flexor carpi ulnaris	e. number of heads of origin
	f. location of origin and insertion
	g. size or shape

G. Label the following two diagrams of the principal skeletal muscles, both anterior and posterior views. Color muscles that are massaged in massage therapy brown.

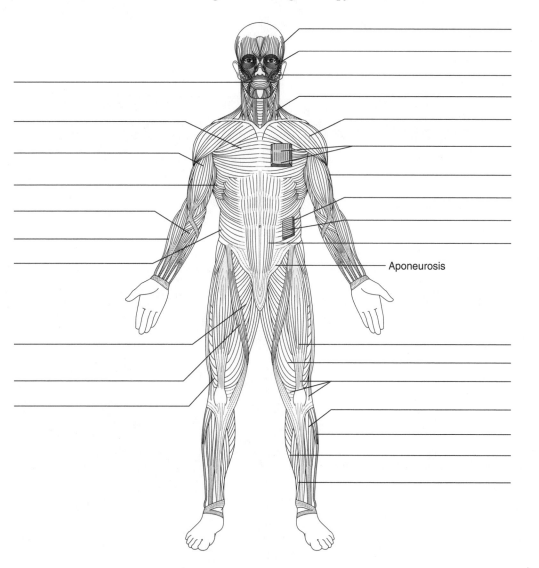

Aponeurosis

Principal skeletal muscles of the body—anterior view

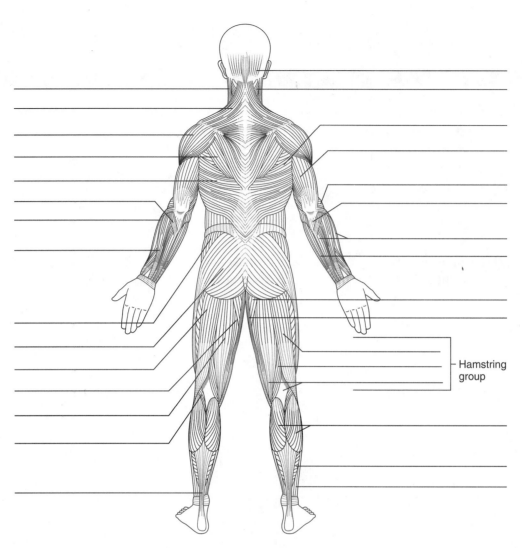

Principal skeletal muscles of the body—posterior view

Hamstring
group

H. Label the muscles of the head and neck. Color all muscles named for location red.

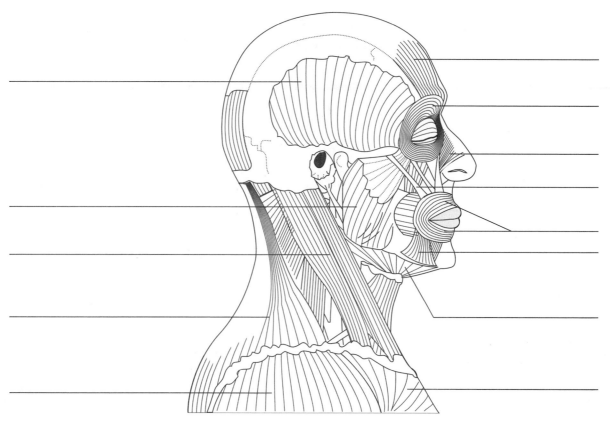

Head and neck muscle arrangement

I. Answer the following riddles by naming the muscle.

WHO AM I?

1. I sit over the eyebrows and wait and see
   if you have a surprise in store for me.

   _____

2. The movie picture gave me a fright, I
   responded with horror to the sight.

   _____

3. A smiling face is where to begin, then I
   can help you laugh and grin.

   _____

4. I protect a delicate structure and faster than a
   wink, if anything comes near it I quickly blink.

   _____

5. This muscle structure opens wide, so food
   and drink can get inside.

   _____

J. Label the following diagram and complete the table.

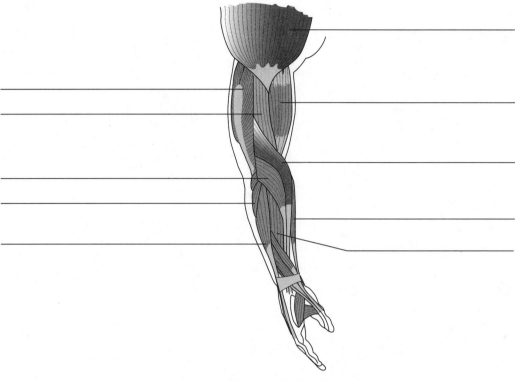

Muscles of the upper extremity

Representative Muscles of the Upper Extremities

Muscle	Location	Function
*Trapezius	A large triangular muscle located on upper surface of back	_____ _____
*Deltoid	_____ _____	Abducts the upper arm
*Pectoralis major	Anterior part of the chest	_____ _____
_____	Anterior chest	Moves scapula forward and helps to raise the arm
*Biceps brachii	Upper arm to radius	_____
*Triceps brachii	_____	Extends the lower arm
_____	Extends from the anterior and posterior forearm to the hand	Moves the hand
Extensor and flexor digitorum muscle groups	_____ _____	Moves the fingers
*Major prime movers		

K. Doing situps can help get the abdomen into shape. Do a situp, and feel the muscles tighten. Label the following diagram with the muscles of the trunk.

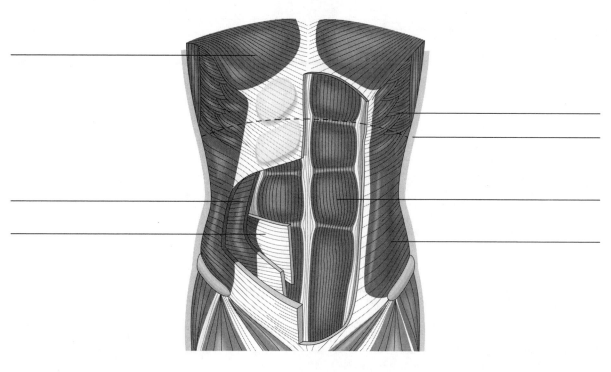

Muscles of the trunk

L. Mark each statement as either true or false. Correct false statements.

_____ 1. The diaphragm is a dome-shaped muscle that separates the thoracic and pelvic cavities.

_____ 2. The intercostals are found between the ribs and help us breathe.

_____ 3. The external oblique flexes the spinal column and compresses the abdominal cavity.

_____ 4. The rectus abdominus is used when doing situps. It compresses the abdomen.

_____ 5. The internal oblique extends the spinal column and compresses the abdomen.

M. Label the following muscles of the lower extremity.

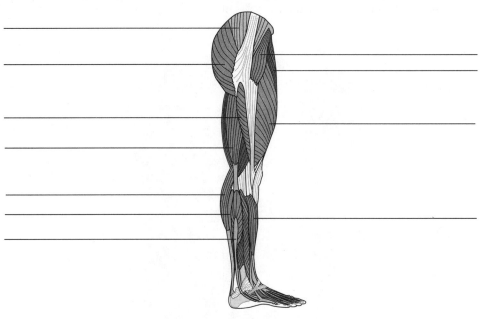

Muscles of the lower extremity

N. Match the muscle function in Column B with the correct lower extremity muscle in Column A. Refer to the previous figure for help.

Column A	Column B
_____ 1. gluteus maximus	a. extends the foot
_____ 2. gluteus medius	b. dorsiflexes the foot
_____ 3. tensor fasciae	c. supports the arches
_____ 4. rectus femoris	d. extends the femur
_____ 5. sartorius	e. abducts and rotates the thigh
_____ 6. tibialis anterior	f. extends the lower leg
_____ 7. gastrocnemius	g. flexes and rotates the thigh and leg
_____ 8. soleus	h. medially rotates the thigh
_____ 9. peroneus	i. points toe and flexes the lower leg

O. Select the letter of the choice that best completes the statement.

1. If you weigh 160 pounds, about how much weight is muscle?
   a. 60 pounds
   b. 70 pounds
   c. 80 pounds
   d. 90 pounds

2. Intercalated disks are found on the:
   a. striated muscle
   b. nonstriated voluntary muscle
   c. nonstriated involuntary muscle
   d. cardiac muscle

3. The characteristic of a muscle to be stretched is known as:
    a. contractility
    b. extensibility
    c. elasticity
    d. excitability

4. Muscles that produce movement in a single direction are:
    a. prime movers
    b. antagonists
    c. synergists
    d. obliques

5. A motor unit is a motor neuron (nerve cell) plus:
    a. one-half of the muscle fibers it stimulates
    b. one-third of the muscle fibers it stimulates
    c. three-fourths of the muscle fibers it stimulates
    d. all of the muscle fibers it stimulates

6. During a muscle contraction, the muscle cell membrane becomes temporarily permeable to:
    a. acetylcholine
    b. sodium
    c. ATP
    d. calcium

7. Muscles are named in a variety of ways; the muscles on the sides of the head are named according to their:
    a. size
    b. location
    c. action
    d. location of origin

8. The group of muscles that make up the hamstrings are:
    a. semitendinosus, biceps femoris, and semimembranous
    b. gluteus maximus, semitendinosus, and biceps femoris
    c. semitendinosus, gracilis, and semimembranous
    d. semitendinosus, biceps femoris, and adductor magnus

9. The effect of training on the muscle can be all of the following except:
    a. improve coordination of all muscles
    b. improve the endocrine system
    c. reduce fat
    d. improve joint movement

10. A tear in the muscle is called a:
    a. strain
    b. sprain
    c. spasm
    d. fracture

P. List three effects of training on muscle efficiency.

_____

_____

_____

Q. Name the major muscle that would probably be worked in massage therapy for the following areas.

1. upper back   _____

2. lower back   _____

3. shoulder   _____

4. forearm   _____

5. chest   _____

6. buttock   _____

7. anterior thigh   _____

8. posterior thigh   _____

9. lateral and proximal thigh _____

10. posterior leg   _____

11. medial thigh   _____

12. lateral leg   _____

R. List one way to prevent each of the following conditions.

1. flat feet   _____

2. tetanus   _____

3. muscle atrophy   _____

4. shin splints   _____

5. flaccid muscles   _____

S. Describe a treatment for each of the following conditions.

1. insomnia   _____

2. fibromyalgia   _____

3. tennis elbow   _____

4. muscle strain   _____

5. rotator cuff injury   _____

6. muscle fatigue   _____

T. Circle the correctly spelled word in each of the following statements.

1. Chiropractors' approach to health care is (holistic, wholistic).

2. The term used to describe muscle pain is (mylagia, myalgia).

3. Muscle (atophy, atrophy) occurs to muscles that are used infrequently.

4. A hiatal hernia occurs when the stomach is pushed through the (diaphram, diaphragm).

5. Tetanus is an (infectious, infectous) disease characterized by continuous spasm of (voluntery, voluntary) muscle.

6. Muscular (dystrophy, distrophy) is a group of diseases in which the muscle cells deteriorate.

7. Lateral epicondylitis, also referred to as tennis elbow, occurs at the bony (prominince, prominence) on the sides of the elbow.

8. Progressive muscular weakness and (paralysis, paralyses) is a symptom of myasthenia gravis.

9. To correct shin splints, choose the correct running shoe that is (confortable, comfortable) and has (proper, propar) arch support.

10. The most common (compliant, complaint) in rotator cuff injury is an (aching, acking) in the top and front of the shoulder.

APPLYING THEORY TO PRACTICE

1. In your own words, describe what happens during a skeletal muscle contraction. How fast does it occur?

_____

2. If you want to get into shape, try this exercise routine. Stretch your arms up over your head. What muscles are you using?

_____

For the buttocks and thighs, bring your right leg up and stretch it way out. Now do the same with the left leg. What group of muscles are you using?

_____

To get physically fit you must exercise every day. Take the stairs, climb a hill, or walk a mile or two.

3. How would you respond to the question, Is massage therapy beneficial? Support your response with at least three facts regarding massage therapy.

_____

_____

4. Mrs. Estelle, age 82, receives physical therapy after breaking her left arm. The physical therapist wants Mrs. Estelle to regain full range of motion in her arm. What group of arm and shoulder muscles will be exercised?

_____

_____

_____

5. Ken is working out at a gym to keep physically fit. His exercise routine involves doing at least 25 situps per session. Name the group of abdominal muscles exercised in doing situps.

_____

_____

_____

6. Carolyn plays tennis at least twice a week. Lately she has been experiencing pain in her right elbow. The doctor diagnoses the condition as tennis elbow. Describe what occurs in this condition. Name other activities that may cause tennis elbow. What treatment will the doctor prescribe for Carolyn?

_____

_____

_____

7. Phil is an active 70-year-old who exercises at least 2 hours each day. He relates to his chiropractor that lately he seems to get tired after exercise and has less energy. As the chiropractor, explain to Phil what changes are occurring in the muscle system as he gets older.

_____

_____

_____

SURF THE NET

Briefly summarize your findings from these web sites, or choose alternate sites for the following topics.

1. For information about muscle contraction, go to http://www.nismat.org/physcor/muscle.html

2. To learn the benefits of exercise, go to http://www.discoverfitness.com/why_exercise.html

3. For updates on sports medicine, go to http://www.sportsmedicine.com/aboutcareers.html

Central Nervous System

OVERVIEW

The **central nervous system** consists of brain, spinal cord, and nerves; its chief function is to coordinate and integrate body activities. The brain is the seat of intellect and reasoning.

Neuron

The structural and functional unit of the nervous system, the neuron has extensions of its cytoplasm called processes or fibers. These fibers are *dendrites*, which carry messages to the cell body, and *axons*, which carry messages away from the cell body.

Axons are covered with a *myelin sheath* called *neurilemma.* The myelin sheath speeds up an impulse as it travels along the axon; it also produces myelin, which protects the axon.

Neuroglia

Another type of nerve cell that insulates, supports, and protects the neuron is the neuroglia.

Characteristics of the Neuron

Irritability is the ability to react when stimulated.
Conductivity is the ability to transmit a stimulus to another point.

Types of Neurons

Sensory or *afferent* neurons carry impulses to the spinal cord and brain.
Motor or *efferent* neurons carry impulses away from the brain and spinal cord to muscles and glands.
Associate, connecting, or *internuncial* neurons carry impulses from one neuron to another.

Function of a Nerve Cell

A nerve cell carries impulses by creating electric charges in a process known as membrane excitability.

Normal resting potential is negative inside the cell, positive outside the cell.

Depolarization is positive inside the cell, negative outside the cell.

Repolarization is negative inside, positive outside.

Refer to the textbook for further information on membrane excitability.

Synapse

A message or impulse going from the axon of one cell to the dendrite of the next cell is called a synapse. The space between is referred to as the *synaptic cleft.* The axon releases a neurotransmitter and the message jumps across the synaptic cleft from one cell to the next.

Nervous System

The nervous system is divided into three parts.

Central: brain and spinal cord

Peripheral: cranial and spinal nerves

Autonomic: peripheral nerves and ganglia, sympathetic and parasympathetic division

Central Nervous System

The **brain** is in the cranial cavity and is protected by the skull and meninges. It is divided into white and gray matter. The **meninges** are the three membranous coverings of the brain and spinal cord:

Dura mater: outer covering of brain and spinal cord

Arachnoid: middle layer

Pia mater: inner covering of the brain and spinal cavity

The **ventricles** of the brain are four lined cavities within the brain that contain the choroid plexus, a rich network of blood vessels that help form the cerebrospinal fluid.

The **cerebrospinal fluid** acts as a shock absorber and a source of nutrients for the brain and spinal cord. A diagnostic test of the cerebrospinal fluid is called *lumbar puncture.*

Parts of the Brain

The **cerebrum** is the largest and highest part of the brain; it is a layer of gray matter that covers the upper and lower surfaces and is divided into two hemispheres. Each hemisphere is divided into frontal, parietal, occipital, and temporal lobes.

The functions of the **cerebral lobe** are as follows:

Frontal lobe is the motor area that controls voluntary muscles; the right hemisphere controls the left side of the body, and the left hemisphere controls the right side of the body. The speech area is located in the left hemisphere.

Parietal lobe is the sensory area that receives and interprets messages from the pain, touch, heat, and cold receptors and helps in determining distances, sizes, and shapes.

Occipital lobe is the visual area controlling eyesight.

Temporal lobe holds the auditory and olfactory areas.

The **diencephalon** is located between the cerebrum and midbrain parts.

The **thalamus** is a relay station from incoming and outgoing nerve impulses.

The **hypothalamus** is the "brain" of the brain, and performs autonomic nervous system control. It is part of the limbic system (emotional control) and stimulates the pituitary to secrete hormones.

The **cerebellum** is located between the cerebrum and behind the pons; it coordinates skeletal muscle activity.

The **brainstem** is made up of the pons, midbrain, and medulla.

The **pons** is a two-way conductive pathway for nerve impulses between the cerebrum, cerebellum, and other areas; it is the center for respiratory control.

The **midbrain** contains the nuclei for the reflex center, which involves vision and hearing.

The **medulla** is the passageway between the brain and spinal cord; it contains the nuclei for vital functions, including heart rate and rate and depth of respiration. The medulla is the center for swallowing and vomiting and vasoconstrictor for blood pressure.

The Spinal Cord

The **spinal cord** begins at the foramen magnum and continues to the second lumbar vertebra. It functions as a reflex center and conductive pathway to and from the brain.

Effects of Aging on the Nervous System

There is a general slowing of nerve conduction due to a decrease in the number of functioning neurons along with the degeneration of existing nerves.

Disorders of the Central Nervous System

Meningitis is inflammation of the lining of the brain and spinal cord.

Encephalitis is inflammation of the brain.

Epilepsy is a seizure disorder of the brain; seizures may be grand mal or petit mal.

Cerebral palsy is a disturbance in voluntary muscular activity caused by brain damage; its main characteristic is spastic paralysis.

Poliomyelitis is rarely seen in the United States; it is a disease of nerve pathways that causes paralysis.

Hydrocephalus is increased volume of cerebrospinal fluid in the ventricles of the brain.

Parkinson's disease shows symptoms of shuffling gait and trembling; it may be caused by a decrease of the neurotransmitter dopamine.

Multiple sclerosis is when the myelin sheath around the axon is destroyed, which slows the nerve impulses; a loss of muscle coordination occurs.

Alzheimer's disease is a progressive disease of mental deterioration that occurs in three stages.

Brain tumors may develop in any area of the brain.

Hematoma is a localized mass of blood collection; it may occur in the spaces between the meninges.

ACTIVITIES

A.   Answer the following questions.

1. List the major functions of the central nervous system.

_____

_____

_____

_____

2. Compare the nervous system and the endocrine system on their roles in coordinating and integrating body activities.

_____

_____

_____

_____

B. Perform the following activities regarding the neuron.

1. Label the following diagram of a neuron.

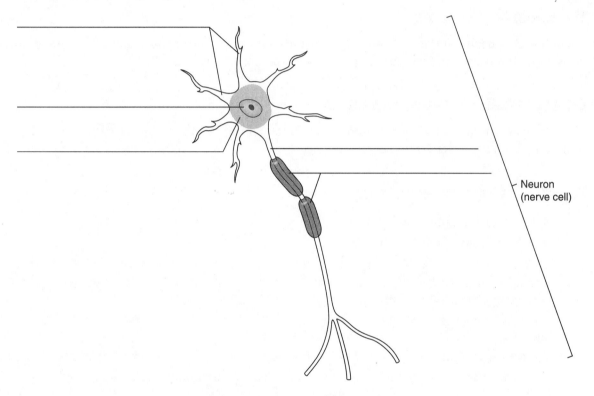

Neuron
(nerve cell)

2. What are the roles of the axon and dendrite?

_____

_____

C. Circle the correct word or words in each of the following statements.

1. The (nodes of Ranvier, neurilemma) are the specialized coverings of the axon.

2. The extension of the neuron that carries the messages away from the nerve cell body is the (axon, dendrite).

3. The type of nervous tissue that insulates and supports the nerve is called "nerve glue" or (neuroglia, neuron).

4. (Conductivity, Irritability) is the ability of a neuron to react to stimuli.

5. Neurons that carry messages to the brain and spinal cord are (afferent, efferent) neurons.

6. A fatty substance called (neurilemma, myelin) protects the axon.

7. The extensions of the neuron that take messages to the cell body are called (axons, dendrites).

8. The two main communication systems of the body are the nervous system and the (endocrine, circulatory) system.

9. The myelin sheath or neurilemma (speeds up, slows down) an impulse as it travels along the axon.

10. Neurons that carry messages from the brain and spinal cord are called motor or (afferent, efferent) neurons.

D. Using the following words and symbols, complete the story on nerve functions.

action potential	ions	polarized
adjacent	K+	positive
channels	large	potassium
cytoplasm	lower	receptors
depolarize	minute	repolarization
electrical	Na+	restores
excitability	negative	reversed
extracellular	open	sodium-potassium
gated	opposite	small
higher	outside	stimuli

A STORY OF HOW A NERVE CELL FUNCTIONS (NERVES-R-US)

In our day-to-day lives we do not stop to think about all the processes going on in that magnificent machine, the body. The heart pumps, blood circulates, and air moves in and out. We jog, talk, reason, and carry out activities of daily living. We will look at just one of these incredible functions.

To understand how impulses (_____) are carried along nerves, we need to know about membrane _____ . Think of the nerve cell membrane as an envelope around the _____ with lots of openings or _____ . Some of these channels are open and allow _____ to move (leak) back and forth inside and _____ during cell activity. Some of these openings are closed and _____ only on special occasions. These closed channels are called _____ . Another special channel is called the sodium potassium pump. It maintains the flow of ions from areas of _____ concentration to _____ and serves to restore the cytoplasm and the _____ fluid to their original states. You may think you have a lot to worry about, but think about the special channel. We have leaky ones that allow ions to flow in and out; we have gated channels that are open only on special occasions and we have the sodium potassium pump.

When the nerve cell is just hanging out, resting, the ions of _____ (potassium) and _____ (sodium) are where they are supposed to be. Inside the nerve cell are _____ amounts of K+ and _____ amounts of Na+. The _____ is true in the extracellular fluid, which has more Na+ ions than K+ ions.

During this time, some K+ cells sneak out through the membrane, which then makes the inside of the nerve cell more _____ . Now we have a situation where the environment inside of the cell is more negative than the environment outside the cell. This state of affairs is called resting membrane potential, and the membrane is said to be _____ .

This is where the fun begins! A sensory receptor picks up a message, a stimulus like a sound, and the stimulus energy is converted to an _____ signal. If it is strong enough, it will _____ a portion of the cell membrane. This is the special occasion that causes those gated channels to open, initiating the _____ _____. The sodium ions in the extracellular fluid line up and march through the gated channel into the cytoplasm. Now the inside of the cell is more _____ . The membrane potential is reversed, and the gates close to additional sodium ions.

Well, just wait a minute. There are too many ions here, so the special potassium gates open and large amounts of potassium leave the cytoplasm of the cell, which results in the _____ of the membrane. To restore order to this mess, the _____–_____ pump gets into the act and _____ the original concentrations of sodium and potassium ions. A simpler way of saying all this is that upon stimulation a nerve cell goes from resting potential to depolarization and then to repolarization and back to resting potential.

Although this action occurs in just one part of the cell membrane, it spreads to _____ membrane regions, continuing away from the original site of the stimulation, and sending messages over the nerves. Your nervous system is an electrical conduction system; sometimes we use such phrases as "sparks are flying." This could really be true. It is hard to imagine that this cycle is completed millions of times in a minute.

E. In the following statements, circle the item that makes the statements correct.

1. A nerve cell has (1, 2, 3) axons.

2. Dendrites carry messages (from, to) the cell body.

3. The first step in nerve cell and muscle cell connection occurs in embryonic development when the nerve cell releases (MuSK, agrin).

4. A (synapse, synaptic) cleft is the area where messages go from the axon of one cell to the dendrite of another.

5. An impulse travels along a (dendrite, axon) to the end where the neurotransmitter is released.

6. The neurotransmitter between muscle cells and nerve cells is (epinephrine, acetylcholine).

F. Match the words in Column A with the related items in Column B.

Column A	Column B
_____ 1. central nervous system	a. ganglia and peripheral nerves
_____ 2. peripheral nervous system	b. 12 pairs
_____ 3. autonomic nervous system	c. cranial and spinal nerves
_____ 4. cranial nerves	d. 31 pairs
_____ 5. spinal nerves	e. brain and spinal cord

G. Label the parts of the brain in the following diagram.

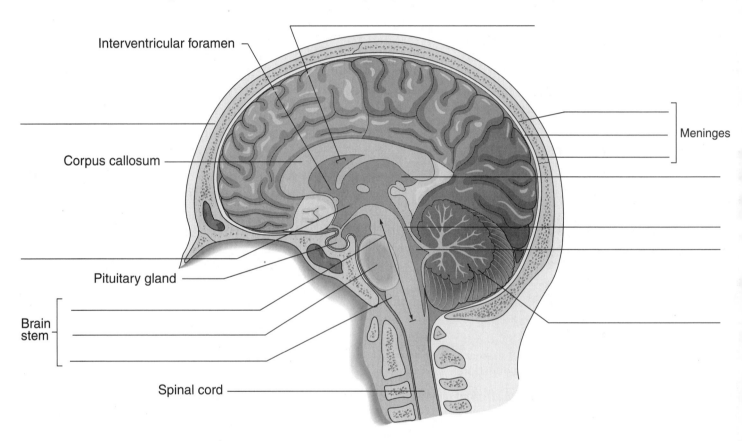

Interventricular foramen

Corpus callosum

Meninges

Pituitary gland

Brain stem

Spinal cord

H. Describe in detail each of the three meninges, including their roles.

_____

_____

_____

_____

_____

_____

_____

_____

I.　　In the following diagram, label the structures for the pathway of the cerebrospinal fluid. State how the path begins and where it goes.

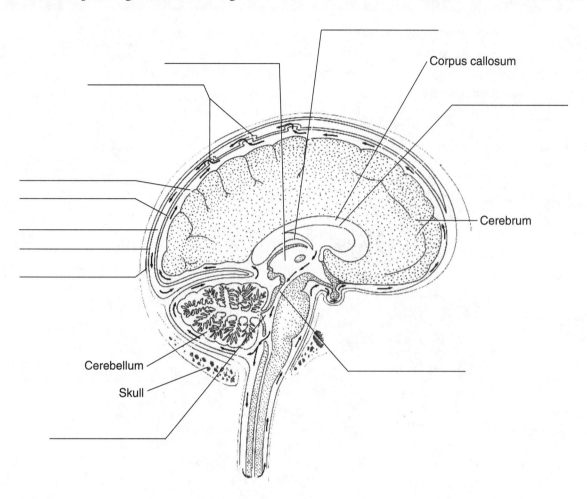

Corpus callosum

Cerebrum

Cerebellum

Skull

J.　　Answer the following questions.

1. Describe the role of the choroid plexus in the blood-brain barrier.

_____

_____

2. What is the function of cerebrospinal fluid?

_____

_____

3. How is cerebrospinal fluid affected by meningitis?

_____

_____

4. What is a lumbar puncture?

_____

_____

K. When you think of a happy time, what comes to mind? How do we know a long slender object with lead on one end and an eraser on the other is a pencil? What creates a memory? What is the role of the hippocampus of the limbic system?

_____

_____

_____

_____

_____

_____

L. Match the descriptions in Column B with the terms in Column A.

Column A	Column B
_____ 1. peripheral nervous system	a. network of blood vessels of the pia mater
_____ 2. limbic system	b. convolution of the cerebrum
_____ 3. layer of gray matter	c. cavities filled with cerebrospinal fluid
_____ 4. dura mater	d. cranial and spinal nerves
_____ 5. corpus callosum	e. conscious thought and responses
_____ 6. choroid plexus	f. inner lining of the brain
_____ 7. gyri	g. unconscious thought
_____ 8. cerebral ventricles	h. thalamus and hypothalamus
_____ 9. diencephalon	i. outer covering of the brain
_____ 10. cerebral cortex	j. band of axonal fibers in cerebrum
	k. outer cranial cortex
	l. occipital lobe

M. Label the lobes of the cerebrum. Color the occipital green, the frontal blue, the temporal orange, and the parietal yellow. Next list the functions of each lobe of the cerebrum.

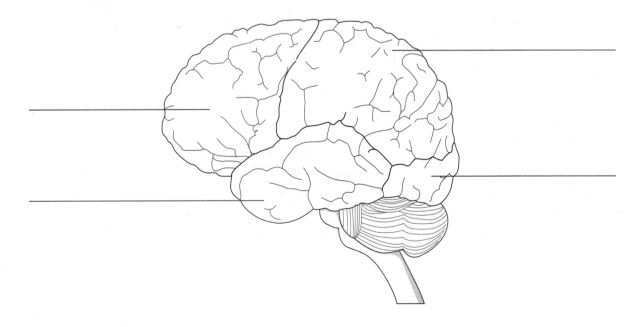

Functions:

_____

_____

_____

_____

N. Mark the statements either true or false. Correct the false statements.

_____ 1. The thalamus receives indirect nerve impulses and relays them to the cortex.

_____ 2. In the medial hypothalamus is the "feeding center," which is stimulated by hunger.

_____ 3. Damage to the thalamus of the brain may result in a total loss of consciousness.

_____ 4. Information relating to skeletal muscle activity is carried to the cerebellum from sensory receptors in the outer ear, eye, and proprioceptors of the skeletal muscle.

_____ 5. The cerebellum is responsible for coordination of muscle movements; raising the hand to the face requires the synchronized action of 50 or more muscles.

_____ 6. The brainstem consists of the midbrain, pons, and medulla.

_____ 7. The brainstem provides a pathway for ascending and descending tracts.

_____ 8. The medulla contains the nuclei for the heart rate and the reflex center for vision and hearing.

_____ 9. The spinal cord begins at the foramen magnum of the parietal bone.

_____ 10. The spinal cord functions as a reflex center and a conduction pathway to and from the brain.

O. Answer the following questions about the hypothalamus.

  1. The hypothalamus is considered the "brain" of the brain. Where is it located?

_____

_____

  2. How are the following systems of the body affected by the hypothalamus?
      a. Autonomic nervous system

_____

_____

_____

      b. Circulatory system

_____

_____

_____

      c. Digestive system

_____

_____

_____

d. Endocrine system

_____

_____

_____

e. Reproductive system

_____

_____

3. How does the hypothalamus affect our emotional states?

_____

_____

_____

P. Complete the following statements regarding the limbic system.

The limbic system encircles the top of the brainstem like a _____ , linking the

_____ _____ and _____ mediates the lower centers

that control the _____ function of the body.

The limbic system plays a role in the _____ of instincts, _____ ,

_____ , and the effects of the moods on _____ behavior. The associa-

tion of good smells with good feelings and the formation of _____ are influenced by

the limbic system.

Q. Select the letter of the choice that best completes the statement.

1. In Parkinson's disease, a person exhibits a shuffling gait, tremors, and muscular rigidity. This disease is thought to be caused by a decrease in:
   a. acetylcholine
   b. dopamine
   c. adrenalin
   d. epinephrine

2. The nerve cell sheaths are destroyed in:
   a. epilepsy
   b. cerebral palsy
   c. meningitis
   d. multiple sclerosis

3. An inflammation of the brain is known as:
   a. meningitis
   b. encephalitis
   c. poliomyelitis
   d. osteomyelitis

4. Epilepsy is characterized by recurring and excessive discharge of neuron activity. Seizures are said to be the result of:
   a. spontaneous, uncontrolled cycles of electrical activity
   b. deliberate, uncontrolled cycles of electrical activity
   c. spontaneous, controlled cycles of electrical activity
   d. uncontrolled cycles of electrical activity

5. A bypass or shunt operation that diverts the cerebrospinal fluid is treatment for:
   a. meningitis
   b. hydrocephalus
   c. encephalitis
   d. cerebral palsy

6. In multiple sclerosis, a symptom called nystagmus is:
   a. a halo around a light
   b. a cataract
   c. tremorous movement of the eye
   d. double vision

7. Cerebral palsy is a disturbance in voluntary muscle action. The most pronounced symptom is spastic paralysis that involves:
   a. both arms
   b. arms and legs on one side of the body
   c. both legs
   d. arms and legs on both sides of the body

8. Alzheimer's disease usually has three stages. The first stage may last from:
   a. 1 to 2 years
   b. 2 to 3 years
   c. 2 to 4 years
   d. 2 to 5 years

9. Aphasia or loss of speech is usually a symptom of the:
   a. first stage of Alzheimer's disease
   b. second stage of Alzheimer's disease
   c. third stage of Alzheimer's disease
   d. fourth stage of Alzheimer's disease

10. A subdural hematoma is a collection of blood between the:
    a. skull and dura mater layer of the brain
    b. dura mater and arachnoid layer of the brain
    c. arachnoid and pia mater layer of the brain
    d. dura mater and pia mater layer of the brain

R. List at least two symptoms and one treatment for the following:

1. Meningitis

_____

_____

2. Encephalitis

_____

_____

3. Epilepsy

_____

_____

4. Cerebral palsy

_____

_____

5. Parkinson's disease

_____

_____

6. Brain tumor

_____

_____

APPLYING THEORY TO PRACTICE

1. Recall your earliest memory. How old were you, and why is the memory significant? Is there a correlation between what we remember and other significant events? Why are commercials repeated over and over?

_____

_____

_____

2. A sign reads, "Fresh-baked cookies." What parts of the brain and limbic system recall the appearance, taste, and smell of cookies?

_____

_____

_____

3. One tragedy suffered by people who are affected by paralysis is the assumption that not only the limbs but also the mind is affected. What is cerebral palsy, and is the mind affected in this disease?

_____

_____

_____

4. A young friend has been complaining of double vision and generalized muscle weakness. Her doctor made a diagnosis of multiple sclerosis. She tells you that the symptoms have disappeared and the doctor must have been mistaken in her diagnosis. Explain to her what is happening and what will happen to her in the years ahead.

_____

_____

_____

5. You see the first stages of Alzheimer's disease in a friend's grandparent. What symptoms occur in the first stages? How long does each stage usually last? What happens in the second and third stages of the disease?

     _____

     _____

     _____

     _____

6. Perform the following nerve impulse calculations: If a nerve impulse travels at 120 meters per second, how many seconds would it take a nerve impulse to travel 900 meters? To travel 360 meters? 1200 meters? 460 meters?

   a. 900 meters   _____

   b. 360 meters   _____

   c. 1200 meters   _____

   d 460 meters   _____

7. Mrs. Randclair, age 82, had a stroke and lost the ability to speak. What lobe of the cerebrum is affected by a stroke?

     _____

8. Dominick is preparing for his final exams to qualify for his EEG certification. He is complaining of a headache, which feels like a dull squeezing pain. What type of headache does Dominick have? Name the other types of headache.

     _____

9. What factor of the aging process interferes most with a person's ability to drive an automobile?

     _____

10. Maria was in an automobile accident and received a severe blow to the back of her head. After a CAT scan was done the doctor reassured the family that the vital function center was not affected by the accident. Where is the vital function center located?

     _____

SURF THE NET

Briefly summarize your findings from the following Internet sites, or choose alternate sites for the following topics.

1. Search for additional information on the brain and its components. Note your findings.

2. For tours of the brain, go to http/www.psycheducation.org/emotion/introduction.htm

3. Search for central nervous disorders discussed in your textbook. What additional information can you find on each?

Peripheral and Autonomic
Nervous Systems

OVERVIEW

The **peripheral nervous system** includes all the nerves of the body (cranial and spinal). A specialized part of the peripheral system is the autonomic nervous system.

Functions of the Peripheral Nervous System

Functions of the peripheral nervous system include:

Controlling the automatic or involuntary activities of the body
Acting as the reflex center of the body

Nerves

A **nerve** is a bundle of nerve fibers, either *sensory* or *motor*. If it contains both types of fibers it is called a *mixed* nerve. A sensory or afferent nerve carries impulses from the sense organs to the brain or spinal cord; a motor or efferent nerve carries impulses from the brain and spinal cord to the muscles or glands.

Cranial and Spinal Nerves

Cranial nerves begin in areas of the brain and are concerned mainly with the action of the head and neck, except for the vagus nerve. There are 12 pairs.

Spinal nerves originate at the spinal cord and go through the openings on the vertebrae; they carry messages to and from the spinal cord, brain, and all parts of the body.

A *plexus* is a network of spinal nerves and veins in a particular part of the body.

Autonomic Nervous System

The autonomic nervous system includes nerves, ganglia, and plexus; its function is to control the involuntary activities of the body. It has two divisions, the sympathetic and parasympathetic. The autonomic nervous system is strongly influenced by emotions.

Sympathetic division is often referred to as the fight-or-flight system. It stimulates the heart, stomach, small intestines, blood vessels, sweat glands, iris of the eye, and bladder.

Parasympathetic division has the opposite effect—to maintain a balance. The most active in this division are the vagus and pelvis nerves.

Reflex Act

The **reflex act** is the simplest type of nervous response; it involves both stimulus and response and is involuntary (reflex).

Stimulus is any change in the environment that causes a response.

Receptors are special structures that pick up stimuli.

Effectors are muscles that react to a stimulus.

The **reflex arc** is the pathway of a reflex action; the simplest type of response, it involves sensory, connecting, and motor neurons.

Disorders of the Peripheral Nervous System

Neuritis is inflammation of a nerve or nerve trunk; symptoms may include pain and paresthesia, which is a tingling, burning, or crawling of the skin.

Sciatica is a type of neuritis that affects the sciatic nerve; pain radiates through the buttocks and behind the knee to the foot.

Neuralgia is a sudden and severe sharp stabbing pain along the pathway of a nerve; types are named according to the nerve affected.

Trigeminal neuralgia involves the fifth cranial nerve; it has sudden onset, with spasms of pain in the cheek and jaw; it is also known as tic douloureux.

Shingles or *herpes zoster* is an acute viral infection, usually on one side of the body, affecting the intercostal nerves.

Carpal tunnel syndrome affects the median nerve and flexor tendons that attach to the bones of the wrist.

Bell's palsy is a condition that involves the seventh cranial nerve; the patient exhibits strokelike characteristics on one side of the face.

ACTIVITIES

A.   Select the word or words from the following list that best describe each statement.

abducens   efferent nerve   peripheral nervous system
afferent nerve   facial   sensory nerve
autonomic nervous system   ganglia   spinal nerves
central nervous system   optic   vagus
cranial nerves   nerve

1. Acts as a reflex center of the body. _____

2. This structure consists of a bundle of nerve fibers enclosed by connective tissue.

    _____

3. A specialized part of the peripheral nervous system that controls the involuntary activities of the vital organs. _____

4. A group of nerve cell bodies. _____

5. The name of this nerve may give you a clue to how it functions. _____

6. The nerve carrying impulses from the sense organs to the brain and spinal cord.

    _____

7. A nerve that carries only sensory fibers. _____

8. This cranial nerve affects the smooth muscle of the stomach. _____

9. This system includes the brain and spinal cord. _____

10. This group of nerves contains mixed nerves. _____

B.   Complete the following table of the cranial nerves.

NUMBER	NAME	FUNCTION
I	Olfactory	
II		Vision, eyesight
III	Oculomotor	
	Trochlear	Movement of eye muscle
V	Trigeminal	
	Abducens	Movement of eye muscle
VII	Facial	
	Vestibulocochlear	Hearing and balance
IX		Movement of throat muscles
X	Vagus	
	Accessory	Movement of neck muscles
XII	Hypoglossal	

C. Complete the riddles, giving the correct name and number of cranial nerves.

WHO AM I?

What is that, what did I hear?
I affect your balance and your ear.

Nerve name and number _____ , _____

I can make your eyes roll and other tricks.
Sometimes one or another of my pairs get me in a fix.

Nerve name and number _____ , _____

I hit the palate and places inside your mouth;
even difficult words I help you pronounce.

Nerve name and number _____ , _____

I turn your head about, going to and fro.
There are times I do not know which way you want to go.

Nerve name and number _____ , _____

When you have a cold, I do not do well;
a running nose really affects my sense of smell.

Nerve name and number _____ , _____

Medicine really does not have a good taste;
I swallow it down quickly in great haste.

Nerve name and number _____ , _____

They say it takes many muscles to cry and to smile,
yet there is only one pair of me to weep and beguile.

Nerve name and number _____ , _____

In this group I am quite out of place,
my action does not affect your head or your face.

Nerve name and number _____ , _____

D. Label the diagram of the spinal nerve plexus and name one major nerve in each plexus.

Major nerve: _____

Major nerve: _____

Major nerve: _____

Major nerve: _____

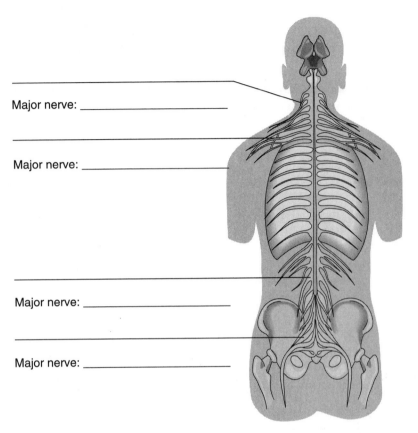

Spinal nerve plexus and important nerves

E. Match the following plexus names with the descriptions.

Brachial (B)
Cervical (C)
Lumbar (L)
Sacral (S)

_____ 1. Supplies nerves to scalp, neck, and part of shoulder and chest

_____ 2. Contains the origin of the phrenic nerve that influences respiration

_____ 3. Forms the median, radial, and axillary nerves

_____ 4. Supplies the posterior of the thigh and most of the leg and foot

_____ 5. Injury prevents normal flexing of the toes

_____ 6. Provides the entire nerve supply for the arm

_____ 7. Forms the sciatic nerve

F. John Smith, age 19, dove off the dock into the water and broke his neck at the area of the brachial plexus.

 1. How would the following functions be affected by this injury?

 Speaking and understanding words

 _____

 Bending his elbow and making a fist with his fingers

 _____

 Breathing

 _____

 Hearing and seeing

 _____

 Picking up his right leg

 _____

 Bladder and bowel function

 _____

 Chewing his food and swallowing

 _____

 Writing a note

 _____

 2. What emotional support will John need to cope with this injury?

 _____

 _____

 3. Name some devices that may be helpful to him.

 _____

 _____

G. Answer the following questions.

 1. Name the two divisions of the autonomic nervous system.

 _____

 _____

 2. List the organs affected by the autonomic nervous system.

 _____

3. Why is the sympathetic nervous system referred to as the fight-or-flight system?

_____

_____

4. What other body system is directly connected to the sympathetic nervous system?

_____

H. Mark the following statements either true or false. Correct any false statements.

_____ 1. Some reflex acts are preceded by a stimulus.

_____ 2. A simple reflex involves a sensory and motor neuron.

_____ 3. Tapping the knee to demonstrate a reflex is a method of checking the condition of the muscular and nervous systems.

_____ 4. The reflex act is conscious and involuntary.

_____ 5. Reflex actions are automatic reactions controlled by the brain.

I. Select the letter of the choice that best completes the statement.

1. The peripheral nervous system consists of:
   a. peripheral nerves and brain
   b. peripheral nerves and spinal cord
   c. peripheral and sensory nerves
   d. brain and sensory nerves

2. The vagus nerve is also known as the:
   a. V cranial nerve
   b. X cranial nerve
   c. VIII cranial nerve
   d. IV cranial nerve

3. The lumbar plexus includes the following nerves:
   a. femoral obturator
   b. phrenic nerve
   c. axillary, median, and radial nerve
   d. sciatic nerve

4. A cranial nerve that carries only sensory fibers is the:
   a. olfactory
   b. oculomotor
   c. trigeminal
   d. glossopharyngeal

5. The autonomic nervous system carries impulses to:
   a. all skeletal muscles
   b. all striated muscle
   c. all smooth muscle
   d. all voluntary muscle

6. A simple reflex is one that has only a(n):
   a. sensory neuron
   b. afferent neuron
   c. efferent neuron
   d. sensory and motor neuron

7. The term *tic douloureux* refers to:
   a. trigeminal neuralgia
   b. Bell's palsy
   c. neuralgia
   d. sciatica

8. In the patient with alcoholism, neuritis usually occurs because of a lack of:
   a. vitamin A
   b. vitamin B
   c. vitamin C
   d. vitamin D

9. The pain due to sciatica radiates:
   a. into the right hip
   b. into the left hip
   c. through the buttock and down the front of the leg
   d. through the buttock and behind the knee

10. The virus that causes shingles also causes:
    a. chickenpox
    b. measles
    c. mumps
    d. hepatitis B

J. Circle the correct word or words in each of the following statements.

1. (Noritis, Neuritis) is an inflammation of a nerve or nerve track in which the patient experiences (paresthesia, parathesia).

2. Treatment for sciatica includes traction and (physiotherapy, physotherapy).

3. A sudden severe pain along the pathway of a nerve is (neuralagia, neuralgia).

4. A condition that involves the fifth (cranial, crenial) nerve is trigeminal (neuralagia, neuralgia).

5. In Bell's palsy, the patient must do (whisling, whistling) exercises to prevent atrophy of the cheek muscle.

6. Bell's palsy affects the (facial, facile) nerve, the mouth droops and the eyelid does not close (properley, properly).

7. Shingles is an acute viral nerve infection characterized by a one-sided inflammation of a (cutaneous, cutanous) nerve.

8. Carpal tunnel syndrome may be caused by repetitive movements in which swelling or (edemma, edema) develops around the carpal tunnel.

9. The diagnostic test for carpal tunnel syndrome is an (electramyograph, electromyograph).

10. The causes of neuritis may be infectious, chemical, or chronic alcoholism. The pain can be (relieved, releived) by (analgesics, anolgesics).

K. Define the word or words and then use them in the crossword puzzle. Definition blanks indicate the number of letters in the answer.

1. Cranial nerve III moves this muscle

    Answer: ___ ___ ___

2. Cranial nerve II

    Answer: ___ ___ ___ ___ ___

3. Olfactory nerve does this

    Answer: ___ ___ ___ ___ ___

4. Efferent nerve

    Answer: ___ ___ ___ ___ ___

5. Spinal nerves and vein network

    Answer: ___ ___ ___ ___ ___ ___

6. Plexus for L4–5 S1–2

    Answer: ___ ___ ___ ___ ___ ___

7. Cranial nerve V function

    Answer: ___ ___ ___ ___ ___ ___ ___

8. Nerve cell bodies

    Answer: ___ ___ ___ ___ ___ ___ ___

9. Stimulates the diaphragm

    Answer: ___ ___ ___ ___ ___ ___ ___

10. Largest nerve in body

    Answer: ___ ___ ___ ___ ___ ___ ___

11. Picks up stimuli

    Answer: ___ ___ ___ ___ ___ ___ ___ ___

12. Herpes zoster

    Answer: ___ ___ ___ ___ ___ ___ ___ ___

13. System that controls involuntary activities

    Answer: ___ ___ ___ ___ ___ ___ ___ ___ ___

14. Painkiller

    Answer: ___ ___ ___ ___ ___ ___ ___ ___

15. Simplest nervous response

    Answer: ___ ___ ___ ___ ___ ___ ___ ___ ___

16. Cranial nerve IV

    Answer: ___ ___ ___ ___ ___ ___ ___ ___

17. Both afferent and efferent fibers

    Answer: ___ ___ ___ ___ ___ ___ ___ ___ ___

18. Motor nerve

    Answer: ___ ___ ___ ___ ___ ___ ___ ___ ___ ___ ___ ___

19. Records muscle electric activity

    Answer: ___ ___ ___ ___ ___ ___ ___ ___ ___ ___ ___ ___ ___

20. Slows the heartbeat

    Answer: ___ ___ ___ ___ ___ ___ ___ ___ ___ ___ ___ ___ ___

21. Involved with hearing and balance

    Answer: ___ ___ ___ ___ ___ ___ ___ ___ ___ ___ ___ ___ ___ ___ ___

22. Affects median nerve and flexor tendons

    Answer: ___ ___ ___ ___ ___ ___ ___ ___ ___ ___ ___ ___ ___ ___ ___ ___

APPLYING THEORY TO PRACTICE

1. When frightened, your sympathetic nervous system reacts. Describe your reaction. How does this affect your body systems? Name one relaxation technique to reduce stress.

   _____

   _____

   _____

2. If your hand touches something hot, what do you do? Explain what is happening.

   _____

   _____

3. A patient visits the doctor's office because when she awoke, her mouth was sagging on one side and her eyelid was drooping. How would you explain this condition and treatments for it?

   _____

   _____

   _____

   _____

4. Your uncle is very worried. His grandson has developed chickenpox and your uncle does not remember having them. He asks you whether he will get chickenpox. What will be your response? Explain about the adult condition caused by the chickenpox virus.

   _____

   _____

   _____

   _____

5. Scotty, age 42, works at a local lumbar yard. One day while at work he experienced difficulty in walking, which was accompanied by pain radiating through his left buttock into his left knee. What diagnosis was made at the company's HMO?

   _____

   _____

   _____

   _____

6. Victoria has been experiencing a sudden, sharp pain on the side of her face that occurs when she is eating. This pain lasts only a few seconds. Victoria visits her dentist because she thinks it may be a problem with her teeth. The dentist tells her that her teeth are fine. The dentist tells her the pain is from what condition?

_____

_____

_____

_____

SURF THE NET

Briefly summarize your findings from these Internet sites, or choose alternate sites for the following topics.

1. For more about cranial nerves, go to
   http://www.faculty.washington.edu/chudler/cranial.html

2. For updates on brain, nerve, and muscle disorders, go to
   http://www.cpmcnet.columbia.edu/texts/guide/toc/toc26.html

Chapter 10

Special Senses

OVERVIEW

Special senses are organs and sensory receptors associated with touch, vision, hearing, taste, and smell.

Sensory receptors are specialized structures found all over the body. A receptor site is stimulated and the impulse is taken to the brain, interpreted, and referred back to the sense. This is called projection of the sensation.

Eye

The eye is a sphere protected by the orbital socket of the skull, eyebrows, eyelids, and eyelashes. The eyes are bathed in tears produced by lacrimal glands. The three layers of the eye are the sclera, choroid, and retina.

Sclera.   The **sclera** is a white fibrous capsule that maintains the shape of the eye; *extrinsic muscles* responsible for moving the eye are attached to the outside of sclera (see Table 10-1 in textbook).

The *cornea* is the circular, clear area in the anterior center of the sclera; it is transparent to let light rays pass through it and is avascular.

Choroid.   The **choroid** is the middle layer of eye, containing blood vessels and nonreflective dark pigment.

Pupil is the circular opening in front of the choroid layer.

Iris is the colored part of the eye. The *intrinsic muscles* of the iris react to the amount of light, *sphincter pupillae muscles* contract the eye in bright light, and *dilator pupillae muscles* dilate the pupils in dim light.

Lens is the crystalline and elastic structure that forms a biconvex shape. The function is to refract or bend light as it passes through. The *suspensory ligaments* hold the lens in place.

Chambers are the areas where the lens is situated, between the anterior and posterior chambers of the eye. The anterior chamber is filled with *aqueous humor;* the posterior chamber is filled with *vitreous humor.* Both substances maintain the shape of the eyeball and refract light.

Retina.　The **retina** is the innermost, third light-sensitive layer, which contains special cells, the *rods* and *cones.*

Rod cells are sensitive to dim light. Cone cells are sensitive to bright light and are responsible for color vision. Within the yellow disk on the retina (macula lutea) is the *fovea centralis,* which contains the cones for color vision.

The *optic disk* or blind spot is the area where the nerve fibers from the retina gather to form the optic nerve; no rods or cones are present.

Pathway of Light.　Images in light "hit" the cornea, then pupil, lens, retina, optic nerve, and finally occipital lobe of the brain for interpretation.

Eye Disorders

Conjunctivitis is a contagious inflammation of the conjunctival membrane; it is commonly known as pink eye.

Glaucoma is excessive interocular pressure that results in damage to the retina and optic nerve.

Cataract is a gradual cloudiness on the lens of the eye.

Macular degeneration is a thinning of the retina area; there is a loss of sharp, central vision.

Detached retina occurs when vitreous fluid contracts as it ages, pulling on the retina and causing a tear.

Sty is a tiny abscess at the base of the eyelid; it can be very painful.

Eye Injuries.　Objects may become embedded in the eye; patch both eyes and get medical attention.

Corneal abrasion—cornea injured; scarring may be the result.

Eye irritations—many causes.

Night blindness—rod cells are affected, making it difficult to see at night.

Color blindness—inability to distinguish colors.

Vision Defects.　Visual problems of the eye include the following:

Presbyopia—lenses lose their elasticity; loss of ability to focus on objects close at hand.

Hyperopia—farsightedness; focal point beyond retina.

Myopia—nearsightedness; focal point in front of retina.

Astigmatism—irregular curvature of cornea or lens.

Strabismus—crosseyes; muscles of the eyeball do not coordinate their action.

Amblyopia—dimness of vision.

Diplopia—blurred vision.

Ear

The ear is a special sense organ adapted to pick up sound waves to send to the auditory center of the brain. The ear is also responsible for balance and equilibrium. It has three parts: outer, middle, and inner ear.

Outer or *external ear* or *pinna* collects sound waves and directs them to the middle ear.

Middle ear is separated from the outer ear by the tympanic membrane; contains the eustachian tube, which connects the ear to the throat.

Inner ear contains the *cochlea* and *semicircular canals.* The cochlea is a spiral-shaped structure containing the organ of hearing (organ of Corti); it picks up sound waves and sends them to the auditory nerve and then to the brain. Semicircular canals are special structures that send impulses regarding balance to the brain.

Pathway of Sound. Sound moves from auditory canal to tympanic membrane to ear bones to cochlear duct to organ of Corti to auditory nerve and to brain.

Pathway of Balance and Equilibrium. A movement of the head reaches receptors in semicircular canals. The impulse moves to vestibular nerve and finally to cerebellum.

Ear Disorders.

Otitis media is inflammation of the middle ear.

Otosclerosis is chronic, progressive disease in which the stirrup becomes spongy and then hardens, resulting in hearing loss.

Tinnitus is ringing or buzzing in the ear.

Presbycusis is deafness due to aging.

Meniére's disease affects semicircular canals, causing vertigo.

Hearing loss can result from exposure to loud noise, conductive loss, and sensorineural damage.

Nose

The nose detects about 10,000 smells; a specialized patch of tissue called the olfactory epithelium has the receptors that send stimuli to the olfactory nerve, which relays them to the limbic system, thalamus, and frontal cortex.

Nose Disorders.

Rhinitis is inflammation of the lining of the nose.

Nasal polyps are growths in the nasal cavity.

Deviated nasal septum is a bend in the cartilage of the nose; may result in a blockage of the air passage.

Tongue

The tongue is a mass of muscle tissue that has structures called *papillae,* which contain the taste buds.

Effects of Aging on the Sensory System

The loss of sensory nerves may lead to a loss of independence and social isolation. There may be a loss of sensory receptors, vision, hearing, smell, and taste.

ACTIVITIES

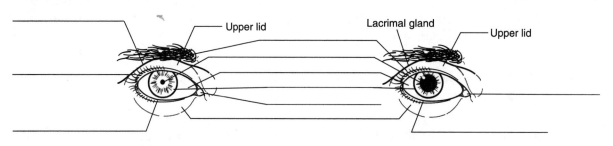

A. In bright light, circular muscles
contract and constrict the pupil.

B. In dim light, the radial muscles
contract and dilate the pupil.

External view of the eye

A.   State how the eye is protected by the following structures.

1. Eyelids

   _____

   _____

2. Tears

   _____

   _____

3. Conjunctiva

   _____

   _____

4. Sebaceous glands

   _____

   _____

B. Perform the following activities related to the eye muscles.

1. Label the diagram of the eye muscles. Color the eye muscle that turns the eye up brown, down orange, to the nose green, and to the sides red.

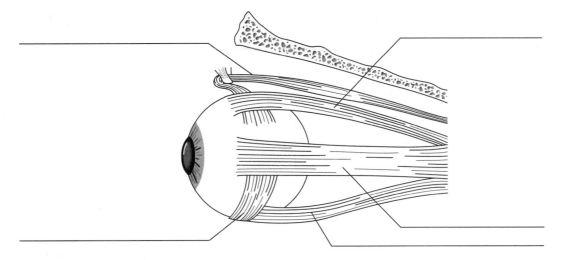

Extrinsic eye muscles

2. How does the name of the eye muscle relate to its action?

_____

_____

C. Complete the sentences using words from the following list. Words may only be used once.

avascular	cornea	optic
biconvex	dim	projection
blind spot	extrinsic	pupil
bright	intrinsic	retina
choroid	iris	rod
color	lacrimal duct	sclera
cone	lacrimal gland	spherical
constrict	lens	temperature
contract	opaque	transparent

1. The sensory receptors for touch, pain, _____, and pressure are found all over the body. The sensation takes place in the brain and is referred back to sensory organs, a characteristic known as _____ of sensation.

2. In the anterior center of the outer layer of the eye is a circular clear area called the _____, which is _____.

3. The structure located behind the pupil is the _____, which has an anterior and posterior convex surface forming a _____ lens.

4. The _____ layer that contains blood vessels has a circular opening in front called the _____, which is surrounded by the colored muscular layer, the _____.

5. The eye is continuously bathed in a fluid secreted by the _____, which flows across the eye and empties into the _____.

6. The movement of the eye is controlled by _____ muscles that are attached to the white of the eye or the _____.

7. Stimulated by a bright light, intrinsic muscles _____ and _____ the pupil.

8. The third layer of the eye, the _____, contains special cells known as the rods and cones.

9. _____ cells are sensitive to _____ light, whereas _____ cells are sensitive to _____ light and _____ vision.

10. The _____ or optic disk is where the nerve fibers from the retina gather to form the _____ nerve; there are no rods or cones present.

D. Label the diagram of the eye.

Ciliary body
and muscle

Path of light

Retinal arteries
and veins

Internal view of the eye

E. Match the following descriptions with the names of the structures in the previous diagram.

1. Curvature of surface in adulthood is convexed   _____

2. Receives nutrients from lymph tissue   _____

3. Watery fluid in anterior chamber of eye   _____

4. Have the intrinsic muscles that control the amount of light entering the pupil

    _____

5. Contains the cones for color vision

    _____

6. Nonreflective pigment preventing light reflection

    _____

7. Tough, fibrous capsule

    _____

8. Jellylike substance that gives eyeball its shape and refracts light

    _____

9. Holds the lens in place

    _____

10. Does not extend to the anterior surface of the eye

    _____

F. Look at an object. Now label the diagram and use it to illustrate the pathway of vision.

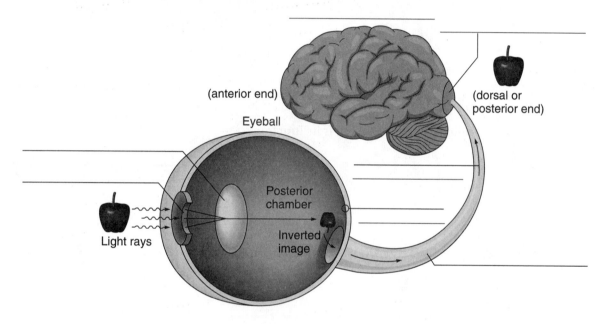

(anterior end)   (dorsal or posterior end)

Eyeball

Posterior chamber

Inverted image

Light rays

Pathway of vision

G. Match the disorders in Column B with the correct description in Column A.

Column A	Column B
_____ 1. blurred vision	a. nystagmus
_____ 2. focal point behind retina	b. myopia
_____ 3. lenses lose their elasticity	c. presbyopia
_____ 4. tremorous movement of the eye	d. strabismus
_____ 5. rod cells are affected	e. color blindness
_____ 6. dimness of vision	f. night blindness
_____ 7. irregular curvature of the lens	g. diplopia
_____ 8. focal point in front of the retina	h. amblyopia
_____ 9. cones are affected	i. astigmatism
_____ 10. muscles do not coordinate their activity	j. hyperopia

H.   Label the diagram of the ear.

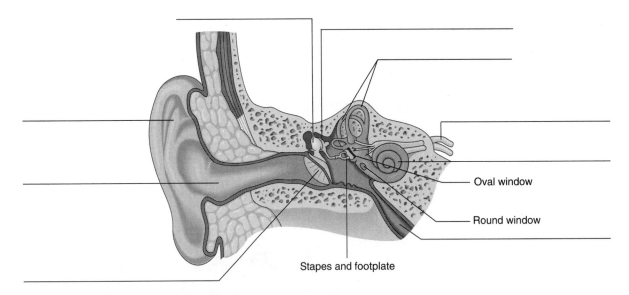

Oval window

Round window

Stapes and footplate

I.   Using the previous diagram, answer the following questions.

1. What lines the auditory canal and what is its function?

_____

_____

_____

2. Name the structure between the outer and middle ear.

_____

3. What is the purpose of the eustachian tube?

_____

_____

_____

4. What are the functions of the hammer (malleus) anvil (incus) and stirrup (stapes)?

_____

_____

_____

5. What is the function of the hairlike cells of the cochlear duct?

_____

_____

_____

6. What is the function of the semicircular canal?

_____

_____

_____

J. Describe the pathway of equilibrium. Refer to Fig 10–13.

_____

_____

_____

K. The hearing process.

1. Listen to your favorite music and think about the hearing process. Using the diagram, label the pathway of sound.

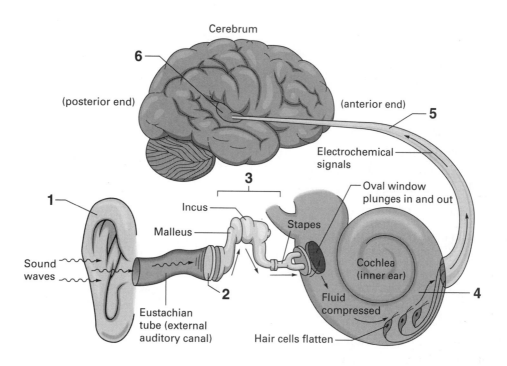

Pathway of hearing

2. Name the structures labeled 1 through 6 in the previous diagram.

1. _____

2. _____

3. _____

4. _____

5. _____

6. _____

L.   Select the letter of the choice that best completes the statement.

1. The ear is adapted to pick up sound waves and transmit them to the auditory center of the brain located in the:

    a. frontal lobe

    b. temporal lobe

    c. occipital lobe

    d. parietal lobe

2. The ear is also involved with equilibrium; the receptors for equilibrium are found in the:

    a. organ of Corti

    b. middle ear

    c. semicircular canals

    d. outer ear

3. The eustachian tube is a connection between the:

    a. outer ear and pharynx

    b. inner ear and pharynx

    c. middle ear and pharynx

    d. inner ear and larynx

4. The special organ of hearing is the:

    a. hammer

    b. anvil

    c. stirrup

    d. cochlea

5. Sound waves are transmitted in the following pattern:

    a. outer ear, tympanic membrane, ear ossicles, cochlea nerve

    b. outer ear, ear ossicles, tympanic membrane, cochlea nerve

    c. outer ear, tympanic membrane, cochlea nerve, ear ossicles

    d. outer ear, cochlea nerve, tympanic membrane, ear ossicles

6. A myringotomy is a procedure done to relieve the symptoms of:

    a. otosclerosis

    b. otitis media

    c. tinnitus

    d. presbycusis

7. Sound is measured in decibels (dB); more than 90 dB for 8 hours may damage your hearing. Ninety dB may be related to:
   a. scream of a jet engine
   b. noise of a shotgun blast
   c. busy city traffic
   d. buzz of a chain saw

8. The main symptom of Meniére's disease is:
   a. vertigo
   b. buildup of fluid
   c. partial deafness
   d. complete deafness

9. A nasal strip across the nose may alleviate the symptoms of:
   a. deviated nasal septum
   b. rhinitis
   c. nasal polyps
   d. sneezing

10. The physician who diagnoses and treats eye disease is called:
    a. optometrist
    b. optician
    c. ophthalmologist
    d. audiologist

M. Use the following words to complete the story on the senses.

astigmatism	presbyopia
auditory	sharp
lenses	smells
nose	taste buds
pain	vision
presbycusis	wax

COMING TO THE SENSES: EFFECTS OF AGING

Once upon a time I could see far and near.
Everything I heard was crisp, loud, and clear.

Now that aging has approached,
I have to ask, "What's that?" as I search and grope.

My eyes have developed _____;
images no longer fall _____ and clear on my cones and rods.

I now need bifocal _____ to see life's smiles and nods.
The bright side of this comes as the mirror you face

Does not show wrinkles appearing, the lines of aging grace.

_____ now causes some eyestrain;

special glasses will relieve the blurred _____ and _____.

Did you say something? I didn't quite hear.

Then again, it may be that I have _____ in my ear.

My hearing loss also could be due to a _____ state;

an _____ aid helps keep my listening skills up to date.

Even though my _____ seems to have gotten a little longer

the _____ do not seem to be any stronger.

There is one sense I truly miss the most:

My fading _____ _____ cannot tell crackers from toast.

The positive side to the fading of the senses you will learn;

I will tell you all about it when my memory returns.

APPLYING THEORY TO PRACTICE

1. Teachers must be alert for an eye condition known as pinkeye. What is the medical term for this condition? What instructions should the school nurse give to parents if a child has this condition?

   _____

   _____

   _____

2. You are asked to give a talk at the senior community center about eye and ear conditions that occur with aging. Include in your discussion glaucoma, cataracts, macular degeneration, presbycusis, and deafness. Describe the latest methods of treating these conditions.

   _____

   _____

   _____

   _____

   _____

   _____

   _____

   _____

   _____

   _____

3. Working in a computer lab at school, your eyes feel gritty and burn. What do you think is the cause? How can this problem be prevented?

_____

_____

_____

4. As you sit in a chair, you start to get drowsy and you feel yourself slipping off the chair. Explain what alerts you to this problem. Describe the pathway of equilibrium.

_____

_____

_____

_____

5. The color of your eyes is determined by the amount of pigment. Explain why the iris is blue, brown, or pink.

_____

_____

_____

_____

6. Richard is an EMT and he arrives at the scene of an accident. Flying glass has apparently injured the victim's eye. Of what emergency procedure must Richard be aware when caring for this victim?

_____

_____

_____

7. While in the chemistry lab, Nichole splashes some chemical solution in her eye. What emergency eye treatment will Marilyn, the school nurse, administer for Nichole when she gets to the health office?

_____

_____

_____

_____

8. Jamal has had chronic ear infections for the past 3 years. The usual antibiotic treatment is not effective. What condition does Jamal have and what will be the course of treatment?

_____

_____

_____

_____

9. Mr. George has been taking aspirin over a number of years for chronic arthritis. He is now complaining of ringing in the ears. What diagnosis may be made for Mr. George's condition and what is the probable cause?

_____

_____

_____

_____

10. Kathleen has chronic problems sleeping and her husband complains she snores loudly. What may be the cause of this problem? Can you suggest a treatment for Kathleen?

_____

_____

_____

_____

SURF THE NET

Briefly summarize your findings from these Internet sites, or choose alternate sites for the following topics.

1. Search for information on color blindness at http://www.encarta.msn.com

2. Explore the computer vision syndrome at http://www.allaboutvision.com/cvs/

3. Learn more about hearing at http://www.jarrettsville.org/myhearing/fr_hearing-testing.html

4. Find comparisons between hearing damage and loud noise at http://www.abelard.org/hear/hear.htm

Endocrine System

OVERVIEW

Glandular systems secrete chemical substances, or hormones, that coordinate and direct activities of target cells and organs. There are two types of systems: exocrine and endocrine.

Exocrine gland secretions go through a duct before reaching their target organs. Their functions are discussed in chapters involving the systems in which they function.

Endocrine gland secretions go directly into the blood stream.

Endocrine Glands

Endocrine glands are ductless glands; hormones are secreted directly into the bloodstream. Glands include *pituitary, thyroid, parathyroid, thymus, adrenal, pancreas, gonads,* and *pineal.*

Hormonal Control. Hormonal control is governed by a negative feedback system or under the control of the nervous system.

Negative feedback occurs when there is a drop in the level of the hormone in the blood; it triggers a chain of events that occurs to increase the amount of hormone in the blood.

Pituitary Gland. The **pituitary gland** or hypophysis is located in the sphenoid bone and has an anterior and posterior portion. It is called the master gland, because it controls the activities of other endocrine glands. It has two lobes.

The **posterior lobe** stores *oxytocin* and *ADH*, which are manufactured in the hypothalamus.

The **anterior lobe** secretes *GH* (growth), *TSH* (thyroid), *ACTH* (adrenal), *FSH* (ovary and testes), *LH* (ovary), *PR* (mammary gland), and *ICSH* (testes).

Thyroid and Parathyroid. Thyroid and parathyroid glands are located in the neck, close to the cricoid cartilage of the larynx (Adam's apple).

The **thyroid gland** is located in the anterior portion of the neck; the thyroid cells are stimulated by TSH of the pituitary to produce T3, T4, and calcitonin. **T3** and **T4** function as *thyroxine,* which controls the rate of metabolism and how cells utilize oxygen, stimulates protein synthesis, stimulates the breakdown of liver glycogen, and stimulates the cellular breakdown of glucose. **Calcitonin** controls the calcium ion concentration in the blood by lowering the blood calcium level.

There are four **parathyroid glands;** they are on the posterior side of the thyroid and produce *parathormone,* which controls the calcium ion concentration in the blood by raising the blood calcium level.

Thymus Gland.   The **thymus gland** is posterior to the sternum and secretes many hormones, one of which is thymosin. **Thymosin** stimulates lymph cells to produce T-lymphocytes, which produce antibodies against certain diseases.

Adrenal Gland.   The **adrenal glands** are located over the top of the kidneys and are divided into two parts, the cortex and medulla. The adrenal cortex produces:

Mineral corticoids, mainly *aldosterone,* which affects the kidney tubule and plays an important role in electrolyte and water balance.

Glucocorticoids, mainly *cortisol* and *cortisone,* which increase the amount of glucose in the blood.

Androgen, a male sex hormone responsible for male characteristics.

Adrenal medulla responds to the sympathetic nervous system and produces epinephrine (adrenaline) and norepinephrine.

Gonads.   **Gonads** or **sex glands** include the ovaries in the female and testes in the male. *Ovaries* secrete estrogen and progesterone necessary for ovulation and female sex characteristics. *Testes* have cells that produce sperm and the testosterone essential for the male sex characteristics.

Pancreas.   The **pancreas** is posterior to the stomach and produces insulin and glucagon. *Insulin* promotes the utilization of glucose in the cells; it is important in protein and fat metabolism. *Glucagon* increases the blood level of glucose.

Pineal Gland.   The **pineal gland** is a pine-shaped organ attached to the third ventricle; it produces melatonin, which causes the body temperature to drop.

Prost-a-glandins.   **Prost-a-glandins** secrete hormones in tissues throughout the body; their activity depends on which tissue secretes them.

Effects of Aging

The production of hormones is reduced as the body ages.

Endocrine System Disorders

Most endocrine system disorders occur because of oversecretion (hyperfunction) or undersecretion (hypofunction) of hormones.

HYPERFUNCTION	HYPOFUNCTION
PITUITARY DISORDERS	
Gigantism: an overgrowth of long bones that occurs in childhood	Dwarfism: occurs in children; body has normal proportions and intelligence is normal
Acromegaly: overdevelopment of bones of face in adults	Diabetes insipidus: a decrease of ADH, causing an excessive loss of water
THYROID DISORDERS	
Hyperthyroidism: increase in thyroxin; symptoms (hypertension, tachycardia, goiter, and exophthalmos)	Hypothyroidism: decrease in thyroxin which slows metabolic processes
	Myxedema: severe form of hypothyroidism that slows body processes to critical condition; occurs in adults
	Cretinism: occurs in children; slows mental and physical development
PARATHYROID DISORDERS	
Kidney stones and bone deformity	Severely diminished calcium levels, which lead to tetany
ADRENAL DISORDERS	
Cushing's syndrome: includes hypertension, muscular weakness, and moon faces	*Addison's* disease: symptoms are bronze skin and electrolyte imbalance
PANCREAS DISORDERS	
Unknown	Diabetes mellitus: hypofunction of the islets of Langerhans, which produce insulin

Diabetes Mellitus.   *Diabetes mellitus* occurs in two types:

Type I—no insulin is produced; occurs mostly in juveniles.

Type II—small or inadequate insulin produced; occurs mainly in adults.

Because of the lack of insulin in diabetes mellitus, cells are unable to obtain glucose, resulting in hyperglycemia. For oxidation to occur, the body must oxidize fats, causing a buildup of ketone bodies, leading to ketoacidotic coma. Patients must be familiar with signs of hypoglycemia and hyperglycemia.

Treatment for Type I diabetes is insulin, exercise, and diet control. Treatment for Type II is oral hypoglycemic agents, exercise, and diet control.

ACTIVITIES

A.   Answer the following questions.

1. Two systems are responsible for coordination of body activities. They are the

    _____ and the _____.

2. Glands that make secretions are composed of _____ tissue.

3. Compare the endocrine and exocrine glands.

_____

_____

_____

_____

B.   Label the glands of the endocrine system.

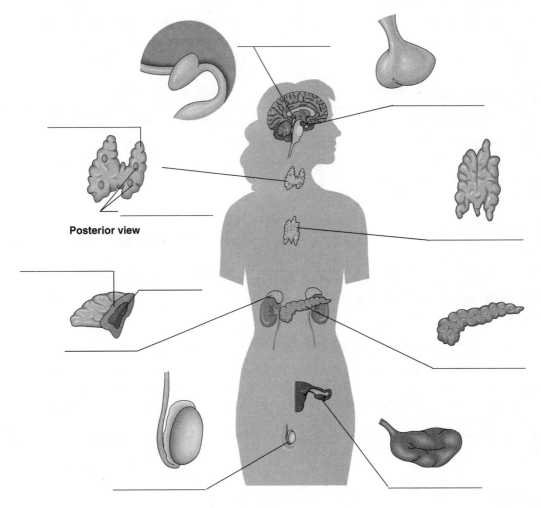

Posterior view

C.   In this exercise, fill in the blanks with the acronyms for the hormones of the pituitary gland.

THE ALPHABET SOUP RHYME

Whether you are short or tall,
the _____ hormone is responsible for all.

_____ helps the cells to produce testosterone,
which changes boys' voices from soprano to baritone.

_____ works on glands that have a neat perch;
they sit over the kidneys and watch the waterworks.

The _____ belongs to the Save-the-Water foundation;
doing its job it prevents dehydration.

_____ stimulates the ovary to produce estrogen;
it also stimulates the testes to produce sperm in men.

The hormone _____ gets progesterone into the act,
which is responsible for keeping the endometrium intact.

D. Negative feedback is a chain of events that occurs to maintain the blood level of a hormone. Complete the following steps relating to glucocorticoid secretion control.

1. The blood level of glucocorticoid falls _____.

2. The _____ of the brain gets the message and sends a releasing factor for _____ to the _____ gland.

3. The gland responds and releases _____.

4. _____ stimulates the adrenal cells to produce glucocorticoid.

5. The blood level of glucocorticoid _____ which in turn inhibits the releasing factor in the brain.

E. Fill in the blanks with the correct gland—either thyroid, parathyroid, or thymus gland.

1. To form hormones of the _____ gland, iodine is required.

2. The _____ is part of the lymphatic and endocrine system.

3. The hormone of the _____ is needed to effect the conversion of glycogen from sources other than sugar.

4. Parathormone is produced by the _____ gland.

5. Heart rate and blood pressure are affected by the secretion of the _____ gland.

6. This hormone produced by _____ decreases calcium in the bones.

7. The lymphoid cells responsible for T-lymphocytes are influenced by the hormone produced by the _____ gland.

8. Calcitonin is produced in the _____ gland.

9. This secretion of the _____ gland helps in protein synthesis.

10. The _____ gland is located posterior to the sternum.

F. Label the following diagram regarding the effects of parathormone and calcitonin.

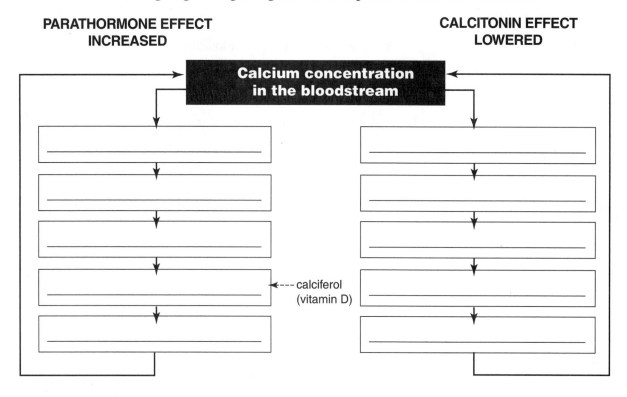

PARATHORMONE EFFECT
INCREASED

CALCITONIN EFFECT
LOWERED

Calcium concentration
in the bloodstream

◄--- calciferol
(vitamin D)

G. Answer the following questions about the adrenal glands.

1. Adrenal glands are located on top of the kidneys. Name the two parts of each gland.

_____

2. Name and describe the functions of the hormones of the adrenal cortex.

a. _____

_____

b. _____

_____

c. _____

_____

3. Next to each statement, write whether it is an effect of **epinephrine** or **norepinephrine** of the adrenal medulla.

a. Dilatation of the iris _____

b. Vasoconstriction of the muscles _____

c. Increases the heart rate _____

d. Raises blood pressure _____

e. Increases blood flow to muscles _____

f. Slight effect on cardiac output _____

H. Mark the following statements either true or false. Correct any false statements.

_____ 1. The pineal gland reacts to the amount of light entering the eye.

_____ 2. The hormone secreted by the pineal gland is melanin.

_____ 3. Light affects the secretion of the pineal; when it is dark, more melatonin is secreted.

_____ 4. The result of the hormone secreted is a drop in body temperature.

_____ 5. The name of the problem associated with dark days or winter is sunshine affective disorder.

I. Compare the following items.

1. Myxedema and cretinism

_____

_____

2. Anterior pituitary and posterior pituitary

_____

_____

3. Adrenal cortex and adrenal medulla

_____

_____

4. Addison's disease and Cushing's syndrome

_____

_____

5. Type I diabetes and type II diabetes

_____

_____

6. Dwarfism and cretinism

_____

_____

J. Circle the correctly spelled words in each of the following statements.

1. Hypersecretion of the pituitary increases GH, which leads to (gigantism, gigiantism), an overgrowth of long bones.

2. In (diabetes insipidus, diabetes insepidus) there is a decrease of ADH, and a person will complain of (polydypsia, polydipia).

3. An increase of GH in adults is called (acromegaly, acramegaly) and results in an overgrowth of the bones of the face, hands, and feet.

4. Hypofunction of the pituitary leads to dwarfism, in which growth of the long bone is (abnormally, abnormaly) decreased.

5. The body of a dwarf is normal (porportion, proportion) and (intelligence, intellegence) is normal.

K. Complete the following word puzzle relating to hyperthyroidism by using the word clues given.

Puzzle	Clue
_ _ _ _ h _ _ _ _ _ _ _ _	1. bulging of the eyeballs
_ _ y _ _ _ _ _ _	2. secretion of the thyroid gland
_ _ _ _ p _ _ _ _ _ _ _	3. increase in sudoriferous gland activity
_ _ _ _ e _ _ _ _ _ _	4. texture becomes rough; tips of phalanges
_ _ _ _ r _ _ _ _	5. people at risk may also have this disorder
_ _ _ _ _ t _ _ _ _ _ _	6. increased blood pressure
_ _ _ h _ _ _ _ _ _	7. increased heart rate
_ _ _ _ y _ _ _ _ _ _ _ _ _ _ _	8. medication used to treat disease
_ r _ _ _ _ _	9. this may develop with disease
_ _ _ _ o _ _ _ _ _	10. sugar in the urine
_ _ _ i _ _ _ _ _ _	11. the type of iodine used in the test
_ _ _ _ _ _ d _ _ _ _ _	12. another name for hyperthyroidism
_ _ i _ _ _	13. enlargement of the thyroid
_ _ _ _ s _ _ _ _ _ _ _ _	14. the cause of hyperthyroidism
_ _ _ _ _ m _ _ _	15. goal is to reduce activity of the thyroid

L. Select the letter of the choice that best completes the statement.

1. In severe hypothyroidism in adults, the condition is known as:
   a. Graves' disease
   b. myxedema
   c. cretinism
   d. Addison's disease

2. Hypothyroidism symptoms include all of the following except:
   a. dry, brittle hair
   b. sweaty and clammy skin
   c. constipation
   d. muscle cramps

3. Hyperfunction of the parathyroid leads to:
   a. kidney stones
   b. tetany
   c. spasms of respiratory muscles
   d. decreased calcium blood levels

4. Hyperfunction of the parathyroid causes the bones to:
   a. develop arthritic changes
   b. become more flexible
   c. become brittle
   d. shorten

5. Hypofunction of the parathyroid leads to the following condition:
   a. myxedema
   b. goiter
   c. tetany
   d. exophthalmos

M. Write **C** if the following conditions refer to Cushing's syndrome or **A** if they refer to Addison's disease.

_____ 1. Hypersecretion of adrenal cortex		_____ 7. Electrolyte imbalance	
_____ 2. Decrease in sodium level in blood		_____ 8. Hirsutism	
_____ 3. Bronze skin		_____ 9. Hypoglycemia	
_____ 4. Moon face		_____ 10. Obesity	
_____ 5. Orthostatic hypotension		_____ 11. More frequent in women	
_____ 6. Hyposecretion of adrenal cortex		_____ 12. Redistribution of body fat	

N. What is the reason for the symptoms polyuria, polydypsia, and polyphagia in type I diabetes mellitus?

_____

_____

_____

_____

O. Complete the following table on the signs of hypoglycemia and hyperglycemia.

Signs of Hypoglycemia and Hyperglycemia

	HYPOGLYCEMIA (↓ BLOOD SUGAR)	HYPERGLYCEMIA (↑ BLOOD SUGAR)
Onset	_____	Slow
Reason	_____	_____
Skin	_____	Flushed, dry, hot No Sweating
Symptoms	Nervous, trembling, confusion, irritable	_____
Breath	_____	_____
Respiration	_____	_____
_____	Little to none	High amount
_____	None	_____
Blood Sugar	_____	_____
Treatment	_____	_____

P. Find the following words related to the endocrine system.

acromegaly
ACTH
Addison's disease
adrenal
adrenalin
androgen
calcitonin
cretinism
Cushing's syndrome
diabetes insipidus
diabetes mellitus
dwarfism
estrogen
exocrine
FSH

GH
gigantism
glucagon
goiter
gonads
hormones
hyperthyroidism
hypothyroidism
ICSH
insulin
LH
melatonin
myxedema
norepinephrine
oxytocin

pancreas
parathormone
parathyroid
pineal
pituitary
PR
progesterone
prostaglandin
testosterone
thymus
thyroid
thyroxin
TSH

```
d h S a i T g p r o g e s t e r o n e g s a t
i y a l n n e o O b W H R K H S T e o u d h p
a p G m r d s m i i O E Z M d p s n m r y t a
b e n f e N r u o t E X O k z a a y e r G H r
e r i J x d z o l r e J y M e d h n o G H N a
t t d h o P e p g i d r c s s t a i t s o u t
e h n n c R q x l e n n i r m l d y l W r Z h
s y a L r y s l y C n d y c e e a a s D m D o
m r l U i A O h q m s a d s a t l E i w o s r
e o g l n l G p W ' c e g i s l i a O Z n H m
l i a a e v F y n r E i P d o g c n t E e T o
l d t e H F n o o s g e w K o r n i i o s C n
i i s n S B s m n a f a x x t n y i t s n A e
t s o i F i e i n B r r y h Y s e h h o m i a
u m r p d g l t y f H t y c q Y a g t s n c n
s P p d a a i r i n o r B h A K y e o a u i o
s K A l n s a s o c o b w F z y h K r r r C n
L H y e m t m g i x c v Z X l E U K k c t a Z
H M r n i W a n i B r Q R i o H S C l K n s p
L d c u E c w n e n o r e t s o t s e t A a e
a J t G u n o r e p i n e p h r i n e m d E p
i i J l F u i O m s i d i o r y h t o p y h c
p E g d i a b e t e s i n s i p i d u s k u q
```

APPLYING THEORY TO PRACTICE

1. It is difficult to imagine that a pea-sized organ affects so many other body activities. If a person had a tumor of the pituitary causing hypersecretion of hormones, what would be the result?

_____

_____

_____

2. You are working in a surgical center; a patient has had a thyroidectomy. Why is there a vial of calcium gluconate at the bedside?

_____

_____

3. Your mother has been diagnosed with hypofunction of the thyroid and is instructed to take thyroxine. What is one of the most important things to remember about this medication?

_____

_____

4. A classroom discussion develops regarding the number of people who will be diagnosed with diabetes mellitus in the next 20 years. The teacher divides the group in two. One group states that more people will be affected; give the rationale. The other group says less; give the rationale.

_____

_____

_____

_____

5. Scientists are investigating the exact role of the thymus gland in our bodies. Where is the thymus gland located? Can the thymus gland be easily found in an adult? Name the hormone secreted by the thymus gland and its function.

_____

_____

_____

_____

6. Mrs. Sanchez comes to the doctor's office and states she is concerned about her son, Carlos, who is 4 years old. He is much shorter than his friends at preschool. Carlos may be examined for the hypofunction of what gland? If a diagnosis of dwarfism is made, how will Carlos be treated?

_____

_____

_____

_____

7. What is the most serious complication of hypofunction of the parathyroid gland?

_____

_____

_____

8. Dave goes to the HMO office complaining of weakness, weight loss, and vomiting. Darci, the medical assistant, notices that Dave's skin appears bronzed. Name the condition Dave may be diagnosed as having. How is this condition treated?

_____

_____

_____

_____

9. Bella, age 17, wants to become an expert swimmer. She hears about using steroids to make her stronger. What advice should the health care worker give Bella regarding the use of steroids?

_____

_____

_____

_____

10. Joy has come to the high school guidance counselor and requests information on a career as a medical assistant. What are the duties of a medical assistant? Is certification required for this position?

_____

_____

_____

_____

SURF THE NET

Briefly summarize your findings from these Internet sites, or choose alternate sites for the following topics.

1. Search for additional information on the endocrine system. Record your findings.

2. For updates on the human growth hormone, use
   http://www.csmngt.com/human_growth_hormone.htm

3. For data on students and steroid use, go to
   http://www.physsportsmed.com/issues/1996/12_96/nb_ster.htm

4. For facts on how to live a diabetic lifestyle, go to. . . http://www.diabetic-lifestyle.com

Chapter

12

Blood

OVERVIEW

The major function of **blood** is to transport fluid throughout the body carrying nutrients and waste products. It also aids in the distribution of heat, helps regulate acid-base balance, and fights infection.

Blood Composition

Blood is made of plasma, red blood cells, white blood cells, and thrombocytes or platelets.

Blood Plasma. Blood plasma is a straw-colored fluid containing 92% water and *plasma proteins.*

Fibrinogen is necessary for blood clotting.
Albumin maintains osmotic pressure.
Globulin synthesizes antibodies (gamma globulin).
Prothrombin helps to coagulate blood.

Blood also contains the following:

Nutrients: glucose, fatty acids, cholesterol, and amino acids
Electrolytes: sodium, chloride, and potassium
Other material: hormones, vitamins, enzymes, and metabolic waste products

Red Blood Cells. Red blood cells or erythrocytes are biconcave cells that have no nucleus and contain hemoglobin. **Hemoglobin** is made from heme (iron) and globin (protein) and carries oxygen and carbon dioxide. **Erythropoiesis** is the manufacture of red blood cells that occurs in the bone marrow. **Hemolysis** is the rupture or bursting of red blood cells. The *normal red blood cell count* is 4.5 to 6.2 million in men and 4.2 to 5.4 million in women.

White Blood Cells. White blood cells or leukocytes protect against infection and injury. The two types of leukocytes are granulocytes and agranulocytes.

Granulocytes have cytoplasmic granules; the three types are neutrophils, eosinophils, and basophils.

Neutrophils perform phagocytosis (the ability to engulf and digest harmful substances).

Eosinophils perform phagocytosis and increase in allergic reactions.

Basophils increase during inflammation and perform phagocytosis.

Agranulocytes have no granules in the cytoplasm; the two types are monocytes and lymphocytes.

Monocytes aid in phagocytosis.

Lymphocytes synthesize and release antibodies formed by the lymph nodes, the B-lymphocytes formed in bone marrow, and the T-lymphocytes formed in the thymus gland.

Leukocyte count is normally 3,200 to 9,800 cells. Leukocytes help protect the body against infection by (1) phagocytosis and destruction of bacteria, (2) synthesis of antibody molecules, (3) cleaning up of cellular remnants after inflammation, and (4) walling off the infected area.

Inflammation occurs when tissues are subjected to physical or chemical trauma or are invaded by pathogenic organisms. The process includes basophils releasing histamine, which is responsible for the increased permeability of the blood vessels, which then allows large amounts of white blood cells through the capillaries to phagocytize and bring antibodies to the site.

The result of inflammation is pus (a fluid filled with dead and live bacteria), white blood cells, and plasma. If the damage is below the skin, an *abscess* may form; if it is above the skin, an *ulcer* may form.

Thrombocytes.   Thrombocytes or platelets are not true cells but pieces of large megakaryocyte cells that help in blood clotting.

Coagulation or **blood clotting** is the process of forming a blood clot that depends on *platelets, thromboplastin, fibrinogen,* and *prothrombin.* Platelets and injured tissue release thromboplastin. The thromboplastin, calcium, and blood clotting factors change prothrombin to thrombin; finally, thrombin changes fibrinogen to fibrin (blood clot).

Thromboplastin also neutralizes the *anticoagulants* in the blood (antithromboplastin and antiprothrombin). *Clotting time* is the time it takes blood to clot (5 to 15 minutes).

Blood Types

Blood types are determined by the presence or absence of an *antigen* (anything that produces an antibody). They are classified as **O, A, B,** or **AB.** The plasma carries the antibodies for these antigens (i.e., a person with type A antigens has type B antibodies).

The **universal donor** is type O, because it carries no antigen; only in an emergency, type O blood can be given to all patients.

The **universal recipient** is AB type. People with this type carry no antibodies in their plasma, so they can receive all four blood types.

Rh Factor.   Rh factor is the presence of another antigen; if you have the antigen you are considered *Rh positive;* if you do not, you are considered *Rh negative.* This situation may present a problem in childbirth: An Rh-negative mother can produce an Rh-positive child, resulting in a condition known as *erythroblastosis fetalis.*

Disorders of the Blood

Anemia is a deficiency in the number or percentage of red blood cells and hemoglobin. Types of anemia include the following:

Hemorrhagic: due to loss of blood

Iron deficiency: inadequate amount of iron in the diet; affects hemoglobin formation

Pernicious: inadequate amount of vitamin B_{12} and intrinsic factor; affects the development of the red blood cells

Aplastic: caused by suppression of the bone marrow by chemical agents, certain drugs, or radiation therapy

Sickle cell: chronic blood disease inherited from both parents; causes abnormal shaping of the red blood cells, which then carry less oxygen and break easily

Cooley's: caused by defect in hemoglobin formation

Polycythemia occurs when too many red blood cells are being formed, causing a thickening in the blood with possible clot formation.

Embolism is a condition in which an embolus is carried by the bloodstream until it reaches an artery too small for passage. An *embolus* may be a blood clot, air, cancer cells, or any other substance foreign to the bloodstream.

Thrombosis is the formation of a blood clot in a blood vessel; it stays in the same place.

Hematoma describes a localized mass of blood in an organ, tissue, or space.

Hemophilia is an inherited disease in which there is a missing blood clotting factor; blood clots slowly or abnormally.

Thrombocytopenia is a decrease in the number of platelets.

Leukemia is a cancerous condition in which there is a great increase in the number of white blood cells.

Septicemia is the term used to describe pathogenic organisms or toxins in the blood.

ACTIVITIES

A. Select the letter of the choice that best completes the statement.

1. The liquid portion of blood called plasma contains water and other substances. The water makeup is what percentage volume of plasma?
   a. 92%
   b. 53%
   c. 55%
   d. 43%

2. An average adult has:
   a. 8 to 10 quarts of blood
   b. 8 to 10 pints of blood
   c. 6 to 8 pints of blood
   d. 6 to 8 quarts of blood

3. Blood does all of the following except:
   a. carry nutrients from digestive tract to cells
   b. secrete hormones
   c. aid in the distribution of heat
   d. regulate the acid-base balance

4. The blood protein fibrinogen is necessary:
   a. to maintain blood osmotic pressure
   b. to carry oxygen and carbon dioxide
   c. to destroy harmful bacteria
   d. for blood clotting

5. The plasma protein that maintains osmotic pressure and volume is:
   a. fibrinogen
   b. prothrombin
   c. albumin
   d. globulin

6. Blood contains the following waste products:
   a. lactic acid, glucose, and urea
   b. lactic acid, urea, and creatine
   c. lactic acid, sodium, and urea
   d. lactic acid, urea, and potassium

7. The white blood cells include all of the following except:
   a. thrombocytes
   b. lymphocytes
   c. monocytes
   d. polymorphonuclear leukocytes

8. Vitamin K is necessary to synthesize the protein:
   a. albumin
   b. globulin
   c. prothrombin
   d. fibrinogen

9. Thrombocytes are also known as:
   a. erythrocytes
   b. lymphocytes
   c. leukocytes
   d. platelets

10. The function of thrombocytes is to:
    a. produce antibodies
    b. carry oxygen and carbon dioxide
    c. create a platelet plug
    d. phagocytize pathogenic bacteria

B. Using the following words, complete the story on the blood.

biconcave	erythropoiesis	heme	oxygen
blood vessel	flat	hemoglobin	protein
bone	folic acid	iron	recycle
carbon dioxide	globin	liver	red marrow
carbon monoxide	heart	lung	short
doughnut	hemacytoblast	nucleus	vitamin B$_{12}$
erythrocyte			

I AM THE RED BLOOD CELL

It is strange that I am called by another name, _____, which has a Greek heritage. The name my family had for me as a baby was _____. I began life in a long (bone) structure, with white walls surrounding me; my special place of development is called _____.

Like any other teenager, as I grew, changes started to take place. First, I moved to another room in the house, called the _____ bones. Sometimes, for privacy, I crawl into another smaller boxlike structure called the _____ bones. I shed my _____ like teens shed baby fat and got a nice new shape, _____. Some people say I look good enough to eat with my _____ shape. To grow big and strong, I have a special food pyramid that includes plenty of _____, _____, _____, cobalt, copper, and a great big helping of _____. I need this since the job description I have to fit is made of two parts, an ironlike substance called _____ and a _____ called _____.

Well, I finally graduated, and now I am armed with my job description, _____, which sticks out all over me like pride. I am now ready to go to work. This whole process of maturation in my case is called _____.

I have applied for a job at the _____ factory, in the circulation division, which means I will be working in these special tubes or _____. My main function is to work as an escort service, picking up _____ from the _____, taking it first to the factory's pump division, then to cells, where it gets dropped off. My next stop is to pick up _____ _____, which has been thrown out of a cell, take it back to the major distribution center, and then to the lungs where it gets blown off.

On my next trip through the tubes, I spot the most attractive molecule, but I had better be careful. My mother has warned me against taking up with that molecule, _____, because it will be a deadly combination.

I work very hard, but my days are numbered—usually I only last about 120 days and then they retire me to the _____ plant, the _____. I will not mind it too much because they recycle most of my parts and *I shall return.*

C. Label the cellular elements of the blood. Color erythrocytes red, granulocytes blue, and agranulocytes pink.

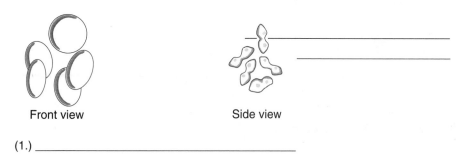

Front view   Side view

(1.) _____

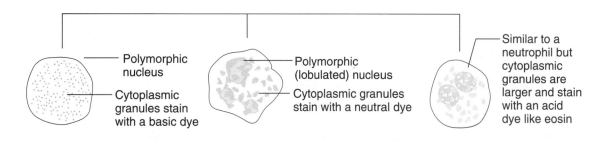

Polymorphic nucleus

Cytoplasmic granules stain with a basic dye

Polymorphic (lobulated) nucleus

Cytoplasmic granules stain with a neutral dye

Similar to a neutrophil but cytoplasmic granules are larger and stain with an acid dye like eosin

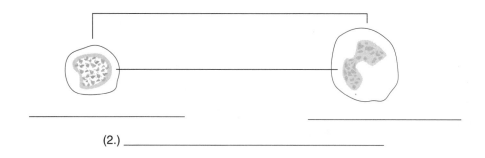

(2.) _____

D. Using the following list of words, fill in the blanks with the name or action of the leukocytes. Words may be used more than once.

allergic	lymph
antibody	lymphocyte
bacteria	monocyte
basophil	neutrophil
diapedesis	neutrophils
eosinophil	pathogenic
heparin	phagocytize
histamine	phil
infection	surround

THE LEUKOCYTE POEM

We are family, and we belong to the leukocyte tree.

The workers are called _____ and _____.
They are so busy at times, they work day and night.

Mono's job is to eat up _____ and _____ them with a wall.
_____ performs an _____ reaction to slay _____,
the round, the short, and the tall.

It is a family tradition to have the young boy's name end in _____.
Their given names are _____, _____, and _____.

The _____ have many lobes and _____,
eating up bacteria and bringing them down to size.

Basophil produces _____ and _____,
which helps fight _____, keeping wounds clean.

_____ pops up all over the place.
When you have an _____ reaction he shows his face.

Most of our family _____ through intercellular space,
leaving not one _____ bacteria in place.

Now come, be our guest, and complete the following table to learn the rest.

E. Complete the following table on the characteristics and functions of the leukocytes.

Characteristics and Functions of the Leukocytes

LEUKOCYTE	WHERE FORMED	TYPE OF NUCLEUS	CYTOPLASM	FUNCTION
Agranular leukocytes 1. _____	_____ _____ _____	_____ spherical _____; may be indented Sharply defined and stains dark blue	Cytoplasm stains a pale blue and contains scattered violet granules	_____ _____ _____
2. _____ (macrophage)	_____ _____ _____	_____ _____ _____	Abundant cytoplasm that stains a gray-blue	_____ _____ _____
Granular leukocytes 1. _____	Formed in bone marrow from neutrophilic myelocytes	_____ _____ _____	Cytoplasm has a pink tinge with very fine granules	_____ _____ _____
2. _____	Formed in bone marrow from eosinophilic myelocytes	Irregularly shaped with two lobes, stains blue, but less deeply than neutrophils	Cytoplasm has a sky blue tinge with many coarse, uniform, round or oval bright red granules	_____ _____ _____
3. _____ (mast cell)	Formed in bone marrow from basophilic myelocytes	_____ _____ _____, stains a light purple and hidden by granules	Cytoplasm has a mauve color with many large deep purple granules	_____ _____ _____

F. Answer the following questions.

1. State the reasons for the process and symptoms of inflammation.

   _____

   _____

   _____

2. Describe the roles of the following in the process of inflammation.
   a. Histamine _____

   _____

   b. Fibrinogen _____

   _____

   c. Neutrophils _____

   _____

   d. Pyrogens _____

   _____

G.   Match the statements in Column B with the words in Column A.

Column A	Column B
_____ 1. pus	a. fever
_____ 2. abscess	b. damaged area below epidermis
_____ 3. pyrexia	c. normal white blood count
_____ 4. leukocytosis	d. temperature control center
_____ 5. leukopenia	e. phagocytosis
_____ 6. ulcer	f. increase in number of neutrophils
_____ 7. hypothalamus	g. liquid containing dead and live bacteria
	h. damaged area on epidermis
	i. decrease in number of white blood cells

H.   Complete the statements by using the following words. Words may be used more than once.

Bleeding	Crust	Prothrombin
Blood clot	Fibrin	Serum
Blood clotting	Fibrinogen	Thrombin
Calcium	Injured tissue	thromboplastin
Coagulation	Liver	

1. A complicated and essential process that depends on thrombocytes is called
   _____ or _____.

2. A cut vessel releases _____, which constricts the blood vessel and stops the
   bleeding. If the cut is deeper, then the process known as coagulation occurs.

3. In the blood clotting or coagulation process,
   a. Thromboplastin is released by _____ _____.
   b. Prothrombin is a plasma protein made in the _____.
   c. Thromboplastin and _____ ions react only in the presence of
   _____ to change _____ to _____.
   d. Thrombin changes _____ to _____.
   e. The _____ threads create a fine, meshlike network over the cut.
   f. The _____ network entraps red blood cells, platelets, and plasma creating
   a _____ _____.
   g. At first, _____ oozes out of the cut; this dries and a
   _____ forms over the fibrin threads, completing the clotting process.

4. What is the role of thromboplastin with anticoagulants?

   _____

   _____

5. Where are prothrombin and fibrinogen manufactured?

_____

_____

I. Multiple choice. Blood tests are ordered by the physician to help diagnose diseases. Circle the normal test results in the following questions.

1. The average number of red blood cells in male adults is:
   a. 4.5–7.2 million
   b. 5.4–6.2 million
   c. 4.5–6.2 million

2. The average adult white blood count is:
   a. 5,000–9,000
   b. 3,200–9,800
   c. 9,000–10,000

3. The average adult platelet count is:
   a. 150,000–350,000
   b. 250,000–450,000
   c. 300,000–400,000

4. Average adult coagulation time is:
   a. 3–5 minutes
   b. 5–15 minutes
   c. 10–15 minutes

5. Average sedimentation rate for adult women is:
   a. 0–20 mm/hour
   b. 10–20 mm/hour
   c. 15–25 mm/hour

6. Average hemoglobin amount for adult men is:
   a. 12–14 g/dl
   b. 14–16 g/dl
   c. 14–18 g/dl

7. Average adult bleeding time is:
   a. 1–3 minutes
   b. 3–5 minutes
   c. 5–7 minutes

J. Answer the following questions.

1. If the hemoglobin in a woman is 25% below normal, what would it be?

_____

2. If the platelet count is 0.20 below normal, what is it?

_____

3. If the total number of white blood cells is 9,600 what is the percentage of the following groups and how many of each would there be?

   a. Lymphocytes _____

   b. Monocytes _____

   c. Granulocytes _____

4. Identify the four major blood groups.

   _____

   _____

5. How is blood type determined?

   _____

   _____

6. What is an agglutinin or antibody?

   _____

   _____

7. What is the possible cause of death in a blood transfusion?

   _____

   _____

8. What is meant by the Rh factor?

   _____

   _____

9. Can a person with type A blood receive type O blood?

   _____

10. Define *universal donor* and *universal recipient.*

   _____

   _____

K. Complete the following table on blood types.

BLOOD TYPE	PERCENT OF US POPULATION	ANTIGEN ON RED BLOOD CELLS	ANTIBODY IN PLASMA	CAN RECEIVE	CAN DONATE TO
_____	41%	_____	_____	_____	A or AB only
_____	12%	_____	_____	_____	
_____	_____	_____	none (universal recipient)	_____	_____
_____	44%	None	A and B	O only	_____

L. Circle the correctly spelled words in the following statements.

1. A decrease in the number of red blood cells and the amount of hemoglobin is called (anemia, anemea).

2. The drop in number of red blood cells is characterized by (parlor, pallor), fatigue, (palpation, palpitation), and dyspnea.

3. The drop in hemoglobin means there is a deficiency of oxygen (transportaion, transportation) to the cells for oxidation.

4. Iron-deficiency anemia may be alleviated by iron (supplyments, supplements) and green leafy (vegetables, vegtables).

5. The anemia caused by lack of vitamin B_{12} and/or the intrinsic factor is (pernicious, prenecious) anemia.

6. Polycythemia, a condition of too many red blood cells, causes (thickening, thickning) of the blood.

7. Embolus, a (foreign, foriegn) substance in the blood vessel, may be air, a blood clot, or another substance.

8. Thrombosis is the formation of blood clots, which may be caused by (mobility, immobility).

9. Hemophilia is a (heriditary, hereditary) disease that interferes with the blood clotting process.

10. (Septicemia, septecemia) is the presence of pathogenic organisms in the bloodstream.

M. Describe the treatment for the following conditions:

a. Hemorrhagic anemia

_____

_____

b. Aplastic anemia

_____

_____

c. Polycythemia

_____

_____

d. Leukemia

_____

_____

e. Sickle cell anemia

_____

_____

APPLYING THEORY TO PRACTICE

1. If a person has liver disease, how would that affect the blood proteins? What other complications could occur?

_____

_____

_____

_____

2. Mrs. Smith's baby is born with erythroblastosis fetalis. The mother is very upset. Explain the condition to her. Can this condition be prevented?

_____

_____

_____

_____

3. In hemophilia, blood factor VIII is missing. How does this interfere with the clotting process?

_____

_____

4. What are the uses for umbilical or cord blood? Do you think the use of cord blood has ethical implications?

_____

_____

_____

_____

5. Kyle is 6 years old and has been hospitalized with a sickle cell anemia episode. Kyle is listless and is complaining of severe pain in his knees. Kyle's parents are worried about his condition. Define sickle cell anemia. What is the cause of his pain? Explain to Kyle's parents about the treatment and the research being done.

_____

_____

6. Estelle, age 82, has been hospitalized for a fractured hip. What type of blood complication can occur because of the immobility?

_____

_____

SURF THE NET

Briefly summarize your findings from these Internet sites, or choose alternate sites for the following topics.

1. Locate the medical effects of carbon monoxide at
   http://www.freenet.msp.mn.us/people/guestb/pubed/cofaq.html

2. Visit the organization Cells for Life Ltd. at http://www.cellsforlife.on.ca

Heart

OVERVIEW

The circulatory system includes the heart, which pumps the blood to all parts of the body and carries away the waste products by means of arteries, capillaries and veins.

Organs of the Circulatory System

Organs of the circulatory system include the heart, arteries, veins, capillaries, lymphatic system, and blood.

Functions of the Circulatory System

Heart is the pump necessary to circulate blood to the body.

Arteries, veins, and *capillaries* are the structures that take blood from the heart to the cells and return blood from the cells back to the heart.

Blood carries oxygen, nutrients, and waste products.

Lymph system returns excess fluid from tissues to general circulation and manufactures lymphocytes.

Major Blood Circuits

General or *systemic* circulation carries blood throughout the body. *Cardiopulmonary* circulation carries blood from heart to lungs and back to heart. For changes in the composition of circulating blood, see Table 13-1 in the textbook.

Anatomy of the Heart

The **heart** is a tough muscle, about the size of a fist, located in the thoracic cavity; the apex of the heart lies on the diaphragm and points toward the left side of the body.

The *structure* of the heart is a hollow, muscular, double pump, with the following layers:

Pericardium: fibrous, double outer layer that has pericardial fluid between the layers

160

Myocardium: cardiac muscle tissue; the wall of the heart

Endocardium: inner lining of the heart

Septum: muscular wall that separates the heart into right and left sides

Structures Leading to and from the Heart. The following passageways help circulate blood through the heart.

Superior and *inferior vena cava* are blood vessels that bring deoxygenated blood to the right atrium.

Pulmonary artery takes deoxygenated blood from the right ventricle to the lungs to exchange carbon dioxide for oxygen.

Pulmonary vein brings oxygenated blood from the lungs to the left atrium.

Aorta takes blood from the left ventricle to the body.

Chambers and Valves. The human heart is divided into four chambers. The four valves within the heart permit blood flow in one direction only.

Upper chambers: right and left atria or auricles

Lower chambers: right and left ventricles

Tricuspid valve: between the right atrium and right ventricle

Bicuspid or *mitral valve:* between the left atrium and left ventricle

Pulmonary semilunar valve: located at the orifice of the pulmonary artery

Aortic semilunar valve: at the orifice of the aorta

Physiology of the Heart

In the *right heart,* blood flows into the right atrium from the superior and inferior vena cava, through the tricuspid valve to the right ventricle, through the pulmonary semilunar valve to the pulmonary artery, which takes blood to the lungs where an exchange of gases—carbon dioxide for oxygen—takes place.

In the *left heart,* blood flows into the left atrium from the pulmonary veins, through the bicuspid valve to the left ventricle, and through the aortic semilunar valve to the aorta.

The *coronary artery* supplies blood to the heart muscle.

Heart Sounds. The valves of the heart make a sound as they close; the lubb-dupp sounds. The lubb sound is heard as the tricuspid and bicuspid valves close, and the dupp sound is heard as the semilunar valves close.

Control of Heart Contractions. The heart muscle is stimulated by specialized conducting cells in the right atrium known as the SA node, or pacemaker of the heart. The SA node sends an electrical impulse to the AV node, which sends an impulse to the conducting fibers in the septum known as the atrioventricular bundle. This impulse divides into a right and left branch, then subdivides into a network spreading through the ventricles called the Purkinje fibers. The electrical impulse continues to the apex of the heart.

Effects of Aging

The heart muscle tissue is replaced with fibrous tissue and cardiac output decreases as one ages.

Disorders of the Heart

Arrhythmia is any change or deviation from the normal heart rhythm.

Bradycardia is a slow heart rate, less than 60 beats per minute.

Tachycardia is a rapid heart rate, more than 100 beats per minute.

Murmurs are a gurgling or hissing sound that can indicate some type of defect in the valves of the heart.

Diagnostic Tests. *Cardiac catherization* is used to determine patency of coronary blood vessels and the efficiency of the structures of the heart.

Stress tests determine the physiological stress of vigorous exercise on the heart.

Infectious Diseases of the Heart

Infectious heart diseases are usually caused by bacteria or a virus.

Pericarditis is inflammation of the outer membrane of the heart.

Myocarditis is inflammation of the muscle of the heart.

Endocarditis is inflammation of the lining of the heart.

Rheumatic heart disease is the result of a strep infection; the antibodies formed to fight the strep infection attack the lining and valves of the heart, especially the bicuspid valve, which leads to scarring and the valve's inability to close properly.

Heart Disease

Coronary artery disease is the narrowing of arteries that supply oxygen and nutrients to the heart. *Angina* is the most important symptom of this disease.

Angina pectoris is severe chest pain; it presents when the heart does not receive adequate oxygen supply.

Myocardial infarction, or MI or heart attack, is caused by a lack of blood supply to the myocardium, possibly due to a thrombus (blood clot).

Heart Failure

Heart failure occurs when the ventricles of the heart contract ineffectively and blood pools in the heart, leading to edema and ascites.

Congestive heart failure is similar to heart failure, but there is edema of the lower extremities also.

Conduction Defects

Conduction defects occur when the electrical conduction of the heart is affected.

Heart block is the interruption of the AV node message from the SA node; there are three types: first degree, second degree, and third degree (or complete) heart block.

Premature contractions occur when the heart sets up an ectopic beat; may be premature atrial contractions, premature junctional contractions, or premature ventricular contractions. The premature ventricular contractions (PVCs) can be benign or deadly.

Fibrillation is when rhythm breaks down and muscle fibers contract without coordination; this disorder is life threatening and can be treated by a defibrillator.

For the **prevention** of heart disease, the National Institute of Health states that lifestyle changes can reduce heart attacks.

Types of Heart Surgery

Angioplasty is a procedure that helps to open clogged vessels; also known as balloon angioplasty.

Coronary bypass is a detouring bypass to allow the blood supply to go around the blocked area of the coronary artery.

Heart transplants are done when an individual's heart can no longer function.

Artificial heart research continues to provide valuable information.

ACTIVITIES

A. Answer the following questions.

1. An analogy is often made between the heart and a pump. What is the rationale for this analogy?

   _____

   _____

   _____

2. Explain the difference between the general circulation and cardiopulmonary circulation.

   _____

   _____

   _____

3. Name the organs of circulation and their functions.

   _____

   _____

   _____

   _____

B. Complete the following table on the changes in the composition of the blood.

ORGANS	BLOOD LOSSES	BLOOD GAINS
Digestive glands	_____ _____ _____ _____	Carbon dioxide
Kidneys	_____ _____ _____	_____ _____
_____	Excess glucose, amino acids, and worn-out red blood cells	_____ _____ _____ _____
Lungs	Carbon dioxide and water	_____
Muscles	_____	_____ _____ _____
_____ _____ _____	Oxygen	_____ _____ _____ _____

C. Select the letter of the choice that best completes the statement.

1. If the blood flow to the brain ceases for 5 to 10 seconds, the muscles will start to twitch convulsively within:
   a. 1 minute
   b. 15 to 20 seconds
   c. 4 to 5 minutes
   d. 6 to 9 minutes

2. As the blood circulates through the body, the blood receives from the muscle system:
   a. carbon dioxide
   b. oxygen
   c. lactic acid and carbon dioxide
   d. glucose and amino acids

3. In the liver, the blood loses:
   a. water, urea, and salt
   b. carbon dioxide and oxygen
   c. glucose and oxygen
   d. glucose, amino acids, and red blood cells

4. The heart is located in the thoracic cavity:
   a. posterior to the sternum and superior to the diaphragm
   b. posterior to the sternum and inferior to the diaphragm
   c. anterior to the sternum and anterior to the vertebrae
   d. inferior to the diaphragm and anterior to the vertebrae

5. The heart pumps 5 quarts per minute. The amount of blood pumped in 1.5 hours is:
   a. 300 quarts
   b. 450 quarts
   c. 600 quarts
   d. 400 quarts

6. To listen to the heart sounds, place the stethoscope between the:
   a. fifth and sixth ribs, middle of left clavicle
   b. fifth and sixth ribs, middle of right clavicle
   c. third and fourth ribs, middle of left clavicle
   d. fourth and fifth ribs, middle of left clavicle

7. The S_1 sound occurs when:
   a. the tricuspid valve opens and the bicuspid valve closes
   b. the semilunar valves close
   c. the tricuspid valve closes and the bicuspid valve opens
   d. both the tricuspid and bicuspid valves close

8. The SA node sends an electrical impulse to the atria causing them to:
   a. rest
   b. depolarize
   c. repolarize
   d. relax

D. Follow the directions regarding each of the structures.

1. Label and describe the layers of the heart and the wall that divides the heart in two. Color layers as follows: outer yellow, middle brown, inner red.

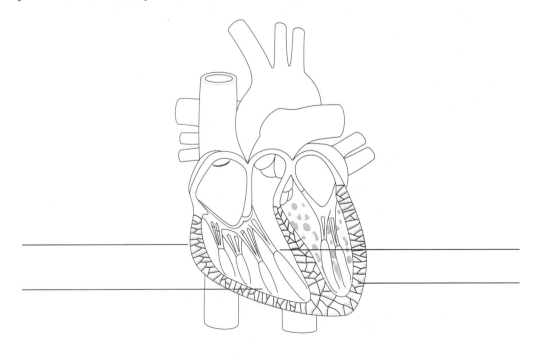

2. What is the name of the fluid between the outer and middle layers? What is its function?

   _____

   _____

3. Label the chambers of the heart. Color the right heart blue (which indicates deoxygenated blood) and the left heart red (denoting oxygenated blood).

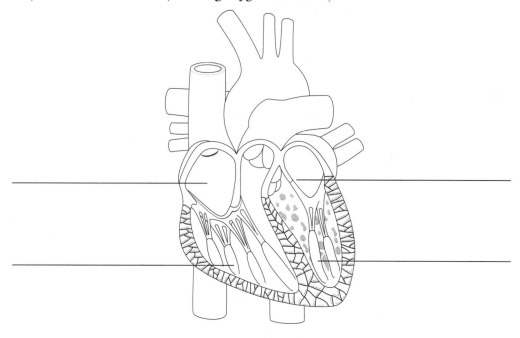

4. Why is the heart colored in this fashion?

   _____

   _____

5. Label the structures leading to and away from the heart. Color correctly those that should be blue and those that should be red.

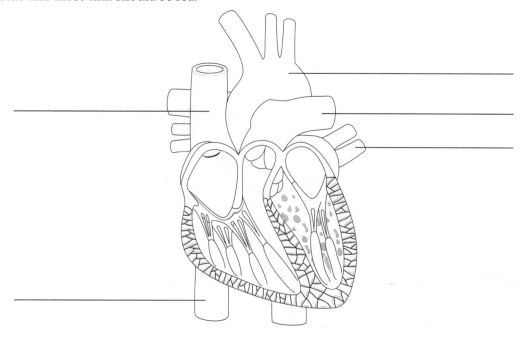

6. Where do these structures go to or come from?

   _____

   _____

7. Label the four valves of the heart.

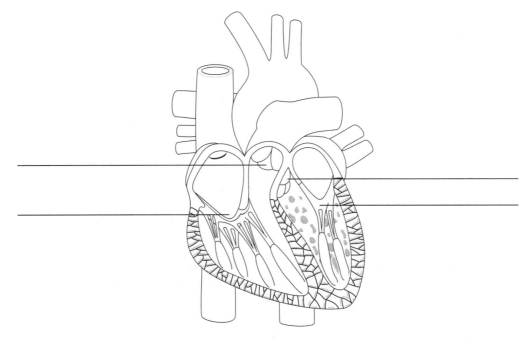

8. What is unique about their structures?

   _____

   _____

9. Where are the valves located?

   _____

   _____

10. What is the major difference between the right heart and the left heart?

   _____

   _____

11. Label the entire heart. Color the structures blue or red according to the type of blood they carry or hold.

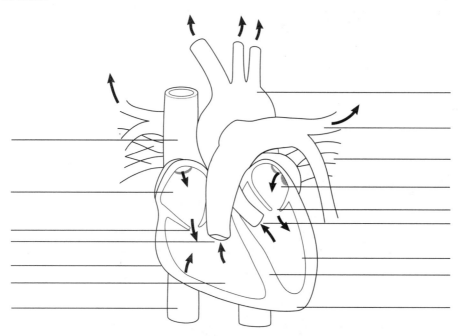

E. Use the words in the following list to complete the story on circulation.

aorta	lung
aortic semilunar	mitre
bicuspid valve	oxygen
carbon dioxide	pulmonary artery
descending aorta	pulmonary semilunar valve
inferior vena cava	pulmonary veins
left atrium	right atrium
left ventricle	right ventricle
liver	tricuspid valve

CIRCULATION OF A RED BLOOD CELL

I am tired. I am a red blood cell that has journeyed through this maze of blood vessels for the past 100 days. I am on my way back to the PUMP factory, carrying with me carbon dioxide thrown out as waste by a muscle cell.

I will be glad to get there to unload this baggage, and then I will pick up oxygen for one of my last trips. The major road from the muscle is called the _____ _____ _____, which goes to the right upper room or _____ _____ at the factory. After getting dumped there, I feel the walls start to vibrate and close around me. I get pushed through a door marked _____, _____. I am now in the lower room called the _____ _____. Just as I get comfortable I hear that same sound again, and these walls start to move from the other side, pushing me upward through another door, which looks like a half moon. This one is called the _____

_____ valve. Now I find myself pushed through the _____ _____ tunnel, which goes from the heart to a spongy-looking building complex with lots of wings; this is known as the _____ factory.

When I arrive I am sent to a small chamber, and there I drop off my _____ _____. "Wait," the supervisor calls out. "You have to take this little fellow _____ back to the PUMP factory with you." As I leave the buildings, I am pointed in the direction of a maze of four highways also known as the _____ _____. I am told that any of those roads will get me back to the PUMP factory.

I choose the least-crowded lane and land back at the PUMP factory on the left side of the building. I am now in the _____ _____ chamber. OH! NO! It is happening all over again. The room starts to shake, the walls start closing in, and my little friend Oxy and I are pushed through a door marked _____ valve. This one has a funny top to it; it looks like a bishop's _____. Now, here I am, in the _____ _____, and before you know it the walls are pushing at me again. Up, up, and away through the _____ _____ valve. Oxy and I are in a bigger tunnel this time; it is called the _____. At the end of this road is a curve with three major arteries coming off it; we will take the road going south, marked _____ _____.

This is my route back to the _____, taking Oxy along. I am so tired of getting pushed and shoved, I think I will just drop Oxy off and stay there and retire to the recycle plant.

Can you guess the name of the pump? _____

F. The following illustrates the action that occurs during the cardiac cycle. Complete the blanks using the words provided. Words may be used more than once.

aorta	contraction	pulmonary artery	semilunar
atria	closed	pulmonary veins	tricuspid
bicuspid	open	relax	ventricles

Depolarization

1. The SA node stimulates the _____ of both _____. Blood flows from the _____ into the _____. The ventricles are relaxed, the _____ _____ valves are _____, and blood cannot enter the _____ _____ and _____.

2. The AV node receives the impulse from the SA node and stimulates the _____ of both _____, which pumps blood into the _____ _____ and _____. The atria are _____, and the _____ and _____ valves are closed.

Repolarization

3. Ventricles, _____, and semilunar valves are _____, which prevents blood from flowing back into the _____. The heart rests.

G. Match the statements in Column B with the terms in Column A.

Column A	Column B
_____ 1. arrhythmia	a. gurgling or hissing sound made by the valves
_____ 2. diuretic	b. difficulty in breathing
_____ 3. bradycardia	c. balloon surgery
_____ 4. murmur	d. pulse rate below 60 beats per minute
_____ 5. mitral valve prolapse	e. inflammation of the heart muscle
_____ 6. angioplasty	f. normal sinus rhythm
_____ 7. pericarditis	g. drug that reduces amount of fluid
_____ 8. dyspnea	h. pulse rate over 100 beats per minute
_____ 9. cardiotonic	i. drug that strengthens the heart
_____ 10. tachycardia	j. change or deviation of the heart rate
	k. inflammation of the outer layer of the heart
	l. may be related to stress

H. Mark the the following statements either true or false. Correct any false statements.

_____ 1. Heart failure occurs when the ventricles of the heart are unable to contract effectively and blood pools in the heart.

_____ 2. If the left ventricle fails in heart failure, edema occurs.

_____ 3. If the right ventricle fails in heart failure, an abnormal accumulation of serous fluid will occur in the abdominal cavity.

_____ 4. In congestive heart failure, there is edema of the lower extremities and treatment is with anticoagulants.

_____ 5. Mitral valve prolapse is due to the improper closing of the valve between the left atria and left ventricle.

_____ 6. A heart block occurs when the conduction system between the SA node and the AV node is disrupted.

_____ 7. First degree heart block is characterized by a pattern of only every second, third, or fourth impulse being conducted to the ventricles.

_____ 8. One form of first degree heart block is characterized by a momentary delay at the SA node before the impulse is transmitted to the ventricles.

_____ 9. Third degree heart block is characterized by no impulse carried over by the SA node.

_____ 10. The atria beat 72 times per minute, while the ventricles contract independently, beating 72 beats per minute; this occurs in third degree heart block.

I. Fill in the blanks.

1. When an area of the heart other than the pacemaker sparks and stimulates a contraction of the myocardium, it is known as an _____ _____.

2. When the atria contract ahead of time, it is a _____ _____ _____ or _____.

3. Premature ventricular contractions (PVCs) originate in the ventricles and cause contractions ahead of the next anticipated beat; they may be _____ or

_____.

4. When the heart rhythm breaks down and the muscle fibers contract at random without coordination, a life-threatening condition exists known as _____.

5. The device used to discharge strong electric current through a patient's heart to shock the SA node to resume its normal rhythm is called a _____.

J. Answer the following questions.

1. Describe the pain that occurs in angina pectoris and myocardial infarction. Are they the same?

_____

_____

_____

2. Name the types of drugs used in the treatment of heart disease.

_____

_____

3. Describe the two types of heart surgery.

_____

_____

_____

4. What is the major problem in heart transplants?

_____

_____

5. What is the action of immunosuppressants?

_____

_____

6. What are the risks involved in taking immunosuppressants?

_____

_____

K. Complete the following word puzzle, using the clues given.

1. Abbreviated term for this condition   M _____
2. Dilates blood vessels   _____ y _____
3. Count should be below 200   _____ o _____
4. Loss of elasticity of arterial walls   _____ c _____
5. Cardiotonic   _____ a _____
6. Another name for myocardial infarction   _____ r _____
7. Lack of this causes condition   _____ d _____
8. Tiredness   _____ i _____
9. Bed rest, oxygen, and medication   _____ a _____
10. Plaque buildup in arterial walls   _____ l _____
11. Therapy to dissolve clots   _____ i _____
12. Severe chest pain   _____ n _____
13. Change this to prevent heart attacks (per NIH)   _____ f _____
14. Blood vessel most involved in this condition   _____ a _____
15. Alleviates pain   _____ r _____
16. Heart muscle   _____ c _____
17. Classification of drugs to strengthen heart   _____ t _____
18. To reduce mortality, provide this type of care   _____ i _____
19. Surgical treatment   _____ o _____
20. Maintain blood pressure and weight   _____ n _____

L. This cryptogram is a message in substitution code. Each letter is substituted for another letter. For example, the letter *k* is substituted for the letter *t*.

Cryptogram for Cardiac Output

SJWMNJS LPKBPK NZ KIH KLKJO ALOPDH LY UOLLM HGHSKHM YWLD KIH IHJWK BHW DNVPKH. NY KIH IHJWK WJKH NZ 80, JOO KIH UOLLM NV KIH ULMR NZ BPDBHM KIWLPCI KIH IHJWK HAHWR DNVPKH.

APPLYING THEORY TO PRACTICE

1. How many quarts of blood are pumped through the heart in a 24-hour period with a heart rate of 72 bpm? If the heart rate was 60 bpm, how much blood would be pumped?

_____

_____

_____

2. Explain what is meant by a double pump.

   _____

   _____

   _____

3. Your grandfather calls and says he is afraid to use his cellular phone because of his pacemaker. First he had to stay away from microwave ovens, now it is cellular phones. How would you respond?

   _____

   _____

4. A 70-year-old woman wants to know how nitroglycerine is going to help her heart. She had heard "nitro" was used as an explosive. Explain the difference to her.

   _____

   _____

5. Explain who would benefit from an implantable pacemaker and/or defibrillator.

   _____

   _____

   _____

   _____

6. Juan Lopez, age 75, complains of chest pain and dyspnea and has a fever. He goes to the ER where a diagnosis of pericarditis is made. Juan asks the doctor to explain pericarditis and how he got this illness. Describe pericarditis and the treatment.

   _____

   _____

7. Maureen Hague notices that her ankles are swollen. In addition, she is short of breath, has a cough, and seems tired most of the time. What heart condition may Maureen have? Describe the condition and the treatment.

   _____

   _____

SURF THE NET

Briefly summarize your findings from these Internet sites, or choose alternate sites for the following topics.

1. For a look at the anatomy of the heart, go to
   http://www.anatome.ncl.ac.uk./tutorials/heart/text/page1.html

2. To study cardiac output, go to http://www.btc.montana.edu/olympics/physiology/defaut.htm

3. To do a circulatory system word search, go to
   http://www.thepotters.com/puzzles/circulatory.html

4. To learn about implanted heart devices, go to
   http://www.content.health.msn.com/content/article/1675.52940

Circulation and Blood Vessels

OVERVIEW

The arteries, capillaries and veins circulate the blood to all parts of the body through the cardiopulmonary and systemic circulation.

Circulation

Circulation occurs through cardiopulmonary and systemic circulation. In *cardiopulmonary circulation*, blood travels from the heart to the lungs and back to the heart. In *systemic circulation*, blood travels from the heart to tissues and back to the heart. Specialized systemic routes are *coronary circulation*, *portal circulation*, and *fetal circulation*.

Cardiopulmonary Circulation.   In **cardiopulmonary circulation**, deoxygenated blood returns to the heart through the superior and inferior vena cava to the right atrium, through the tricuspid valve to the right ventricle, through the pulmonary semilunar valve to the pulmonary artery and finally to the lungs.

The gaseous exchange between carbon dioxide and oxygen takes place in the lungs. Oxygenated blood returns from the lungs through the pulmonary veins to the left atrium, through the bicuspid valve to the left ventricle, through the aortic semilunar valve to the aorta, and to all parts of the body.

Path of General Circulation.   The *aorta*, the largest artery in the body, emerges from the heart and its first branch. The coronary artery goes to the heart and then forms the *aortic arch*. Three arterial branches from the aortic arch are the brachiocephalic, the left common carotid, and the left subclavian arteries. The aortic arch descends and many arteries branch from it; for example, they go to the chest, organs of digestion, reproductive organs, and the rest of the body.

Coronary Circulation.   Two branches of the coronary artery, right and left, come from the aorta. Their branches feed the muscles of the heart. Blood returns to the right atrium through the *coronary sinus* into which the coronary veins empty.

Portal Circulation.   Portal circulation is a specialized circulation in which veins from the pancreas, stomach, small intestine, spleen, and colon empty into and form the *portal vein*. The portal vein carries blood to the liver, and glucose gets stored as glycogen. After going through the liver, the blood leaves through the *hepatic vein* to the inferior vena cava.

Fetal Circulation. In the fetus, the placenta acts like the lungs and therefore cardiopulmonary circulation is not necessary. Specialized structures that enable the blood to bypass the lungs are the *foramen ovale*, an opening between the right atrium and the left atrium, and the *ductus arteriosus*, a structure between the pulmonary artery and the aorta. The structures usually close after birth.

Blood Vessels

Blood vessels include the arteries, capillaries, and veins. The **artery** has an elastic, muscular, thick wall that carries oxygenated blood (except for the pulmonary artery). It has three layers:

> *Tunica adventitia:* outer layer; fibrous connective tissue with smooth muscle that gives it elasticity
>
> *Tunica media:* middle layer; muscle cells arranged in a circular fashion enable the vessels to dilate and constrict
>
> *Tunica interna:* inner lining; smooth and shiny

Capillaries are the thinnest vessels; they connect the arteries and the veins. The exchange of gases and nutrients takes place in the capillaries.

Veins carry deoxygenated blood to the heart (except for the pulmonary veins). This structure is similar to that of arteries, but the three layers are thinner. Within the veins are valves that prevent the backflow of blood.

The valves help push blood back to the heart. In addition, the skeletal muscles contracting and the action of the diaphragm during respiration assist in the *venous return.*

Effects of Aging

Arteries are less elastic and the heart has to work harder to push the blood through the arteries as the body ages. Researchers believe normal blood pressure for older persons may be 140/90.

Blood Pressure

Blood pressure is the pressure of the blood against the arterial walls when the heart contracts (*systolic*) and relaxes (*diastolic*). Blood pressure is recorded with the systolic number on top and the diastolic number on bottom. A normal blood pressure is 120/80. The difference between the systole and the diastole is the *pulse pressure.*

Pulse

Pulse is the alternating expansion and contraction of an artery as the blood flows through it. The rate is usually the same as the heart. The pulse points are the temporal, carotid, brachial, radial, femoral, popliteal, and dorsalis pedis.

Congenital Heart Defects

Congenital heart defects occur when there is a malformation of the heart. *Cyanosis* is usually the first sign of a problem.

Disorders of the Blood Vessels

> *Aneurysm* is a ballooning of the arterial wall.
>
> *Arteriosclerosis* is when arterial walls thicken because of a loss of elasticity.

Atherosclerosis is a deposit of fatty substances that forms along the arterial wall.

Gangrene is death of body tissue due to an insufficient blood supply.

Phlebitis is inflammation of the lining of a vein.

Embolism is a traveling blood clot.

Varicose veins are swollen veins.

Hemorrhoids are varicose veins of the rectum.

Cerebral hemorrhage is bleeding from blood vessels within the brain.

Peripheral vascular disease (PVD) is caused by a blockage in the arteries, usually in the legs. *Claudication* is a cramping pain in the legs or buttocks that occurs when walking is a primary symptom.

Hypertension is high blood pressure. It is called the "silent killer," because it has no symptoms. It leads to strokes, heart attacks, and kidney failure.

Transient ischemic attacks are temporary interruptions of the blood flow to the brain. Of people with transient ischemic attacks, 50% have a major stroke within the following year.

Cerebrovascular accident (CVA), or stroke, is the sudden interruption of blood to the brain. Symptoms depend on which side of the brain has its blood supply interrupted.

ACTIVITIES

A.　Answer the following questions relating to circulation.

1. Name the two major circulatory systems.

　_____

2. Describe the three specialized systemic routes.

　_____

　_____

　_____

3. Describe coronary circulation.

　_____

　_____

4. What special structure is on the posterior wall of the right atrium?

　_____

5. In portal circulation, which veins form the portal vein?

　_____

6. Is arterial circulation related to portal circulation?

　_____

7. The blood in the portal vein goes to the liver. What is the effect of the liver on the following?
   a. Glucose and blood glucose concentration

   _____

   b. Amino acids

   _____

8. Blood leaves the liver through what vein?

   _____

9. Fetal circulation is the unique circulation between mother and developing fetus. What is the difference between the fetal heart and the adult heart? Where does the exchange of gases take place?

   _____

   _____

10. What is the purpose of the following?
    a. Foramen ovale

    _____

    b. Ductus arteriosus

    _____

B. Fill in the blanks to complete the following statements.

1. After the blood goes through the cardiopulmonary circulation, the blood then goes to the major artery, the _____.

2. The first branch is the _____ artery, which takes blood to the _____. The aorta now forms an arch.

3. The right branch off the aortic arch is the _____ artery, which subdivides into the _____ artery to the shoulder and the _____ _____ artery to the _____ and _____.

4. The left branch off the aortic arch has two arteries, the left _____ _____ artery to the _____ and _____ and the subclavian artery to the _____.

5. The arch turns downward and is called the descending aorta with the following arteries coming off as branches: the _____ artery to the chest cavity and the celiac artery to the _____, _____, _____, and _____.

C. Select the letter of the choice that best completes the statement.

1. The pulmonary artery carries deoxygenated blood from the:
    a. right atrium to the lungs
    b. right ventricle to the lungs
    c. lungs to the left atrium
    d. left ventricle to all parts of the body

2. The outer layer of the arteries is the:
    a. tunica adventitia
    b. tunica media
    c. tunica interna
    d. tunica intima

3. The ability of the arteries to withstand a sudden large increase in pressure is accomplished by the:
    a. elasticity of the smooth muscles
    b. muscle cells arranged in a circular pattern
    c. smooth lining of the tunica interna
    d. tunica media

4. The arteries' ability to dilate and constrict is accomplished by:
    a. elasticity of the smooth muscles
    b. muscle cells arranged in a circular pattern
    c. smooth lining of tunica interna
    d. tunica externa

5. The capillaries are branches of the:
    a. metarterioles
    b. metavenuoles
    c. arterioles
    d. venules

6. The thinnest of the capillary walls allows:
    a. only oxygen out of the capillary
    b. only metabolic wastes out of the capillary
    c. only nitrogenous material out of the capillary
    d. only oxygen, metabolic wastes, nitrogenous material, and carbon dioxide out of the capillary

7. Blood flow through the capillaries is controlled by the:
    a. smooth muscles of adventitia
    b. precapillary sphincters
    c. circular muscles in the media
    d. skeletal muscles

8. The major structural difference between arteries and veins is that in the veins, the:
    a. walls are thicker
    b. valves are present
    c. walls are the same, valves are present
    d. walls are thinner, valves are present

9. The contractions of skeletal muscle:
   a. help capillaries circulate blood
   b. assist in venous return
   c. assist in arterial distribution
   d. have no role in circulation

10. All of the following activities assist in the circulation of blood except:
    a. walking for 30 minutes
    b. running for 5 minutes
    c. sitting at a computer
    d. gardening

D. Answer the following riddles, using the arteries from the list.

brachial	external carotid	popliteal
celiac	femoral	radial
common iliac	internal carotid	vertebral
dorsal pedalis		

WHO AM I?

1. I run up and down the back
   bringing blood to the central nervous system track.   _____

2. You feel me often at your wrist,
   running or jumping gives my numbers a lift.   _____

3. I struggle to get to all the parts of the brain,
   where intelligence and coordination reign.   _____

4. I run down and through the upper bone,
   get cuffed around, please leave me alone!   _____

5. They call me common, I go from place to place;
   I branch down the legs and into the pelvic space.   _____

6. I am really at the end of the line.
   My companion vein has an upward climb.   _____

7. If you reach down behind your knee,
   check around and you are sure to feel me.   _____

8. When you get embarrassed and your face turns red,
   my vessels have dilated, up to the hair roots on your head. _____

9. I am hungry for nutrients from the food intake;
   I am now undecided, which of the four roads should I take?   _____

10. I sometimes get plugged and blood does not get through;
    the legs and the feet do not know what to do.   _____

E. Label the arteries in the following diagram.

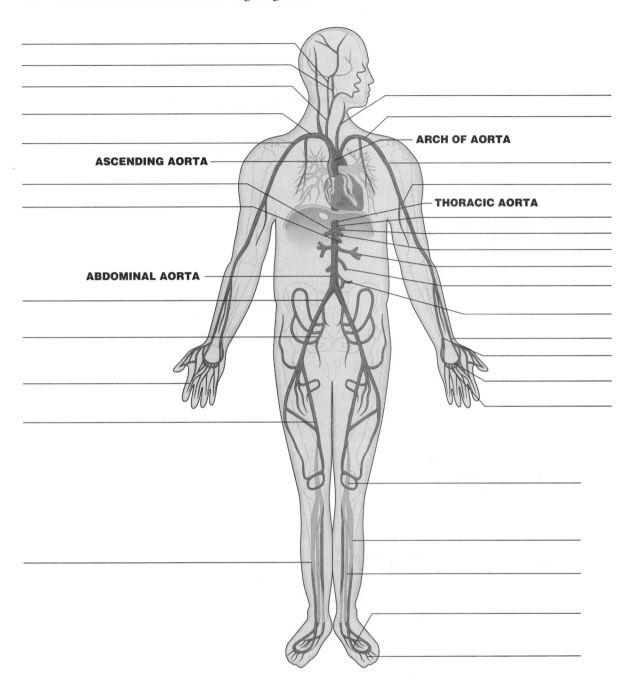

ARCH OF AORTA

ASCENDING AORTA

THORACIC AORTA

ABDOMINAL AORTA

F. Label the diagram of the different types of blood vessels and their layers. Color the arteries red, the veins blue, and the capillaries yellow.

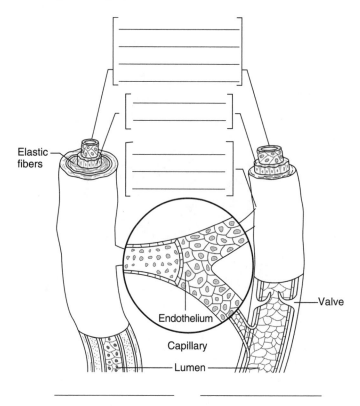

Elastic fibers

Valve

Endothelium

Capillary

Lumen

(A) Types of blood vessels and their general structure

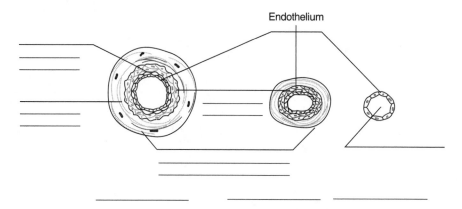

Endothelium

(B) Cross section of blood vessels

G. Label the veins in the following diagram.

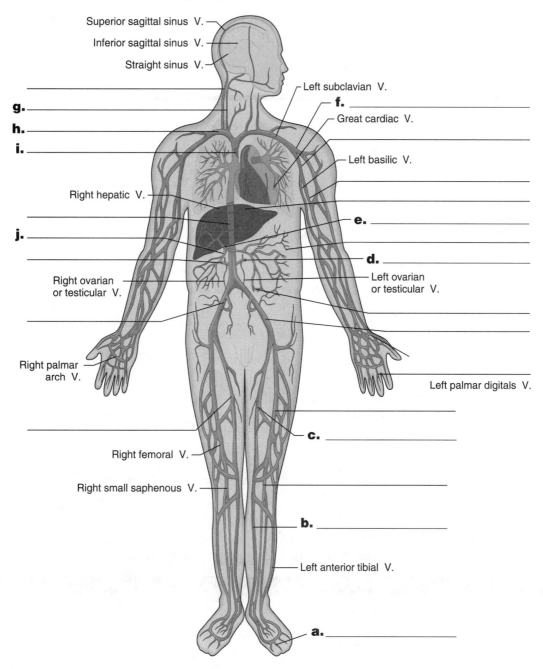

Superior sagittal sinus V.
Inferior sagittal sinus V.
Straight sinus V.

g.
h.
i.

Right hepatic V.

j.

Right ovarian
or testicular V.

Right palmar
arch V.

Right femoral V.

Right small saphenous V.

Left subclavian V.
f.
Great cardiac V.

Left basilic V.

e.

d.

Left ovarian
or testicular V.

Left palmar digitals V.

c.

b.

Left anterior tibial V.

a.

H. Using the labels from the previous diagram, match the correct letter with each statement.

_____ 1. Affected in varicose veins

_____ 2. Furthest branch in feet

_____ 3. Largest vein in body

_____ 4. From the kidney

_____ 5. Returns blood to the right atrium

_____ 6. Branches into the shoulder and axilla

_____ 7. Involved in portal circulation

_____ 8. Branches into external and internal jugular

_____ 9. Blood from small intestine and colon

_____ 10. Blood from brain to superior vena cava

I. Fill in the blanks to complete the statements on blood pressure and pulse.

1. The pressure measured as the heart contracts is the _____ pressure; the pressure measured as the heart relaxes is the _____ pressure.

2. Pulse measures the alternating _____ and _____ of an artery as blood flows through it.

3. Pulse rate is usually the same as the _____ rate.

J. Answer the following questions.

1. Take the blood pressures of two of your classmates. Record the data.

   _____

   _____

2. Are they within normal range?

   _____

3. What is pulse pressure?

   _____

   _____

K. The following questions relate to pulse points.

1. Take your pulse at the following pulse sites and describe their locations.

Pulse Point	Rate	Location
Temporal	_____	_____
Carotid	_____	_____
Brachial	_____	_____
Radial	_____	_____
Popliteal	_____	_____
Dorsalis pedis	_____	_____

2. Is there a difference in any of your readings?

   _____

3. Which is the most difficult or faintest pulse point?

   _____

   _____

L. Match the disorder in Column A with the explanation in Column B

Column A	Column B
_____ 1. aneurysm	a. cramping in buttocks while walking
_____ 2. phlebitis	b. bleeding in blood vessels in brain
_____ 3. hemorrhoids	c. fatty buildup in artery
_____ 4. cerebral hemorrhage	d. ballooning of an artery
_____ 5. varicose veins	e. inflammation of veins
_____ 6. embolism	f. bluish discoloration in skin
_____ 7. peripheral vascular disease (PVD)	g. death of body tissue
_____ 8. claudication	h. traveling blood clot
_____ 9. cyanosis	i. varicose veins in the walls of the rectum
_____ 10. gangrene	j. swollen veins
	k. loss of elasticity
	l. blockage of artery in legs

M. Compare the following pairs.

1. Arteriole/venule

   _____

   _____

2. Phlebitis/thrombosis

   _____

   _____

3. Ischemia/gangrene

   _____

   _____

4. Embolism/thrombus

   _____

   _____

5. Transient ischemic attack/stroke

   _____

   _____

N.   Label the diagram of affected sites and resulting complications of atherosclerosis. Which arteries are involved in the following?

1. Stroke _____

2. Angina _____

3. Aneurysm _____

4. Hypertension _____

5. Peripheral vascular disease _____

AFFECTED SITE   **COMPLICATION**

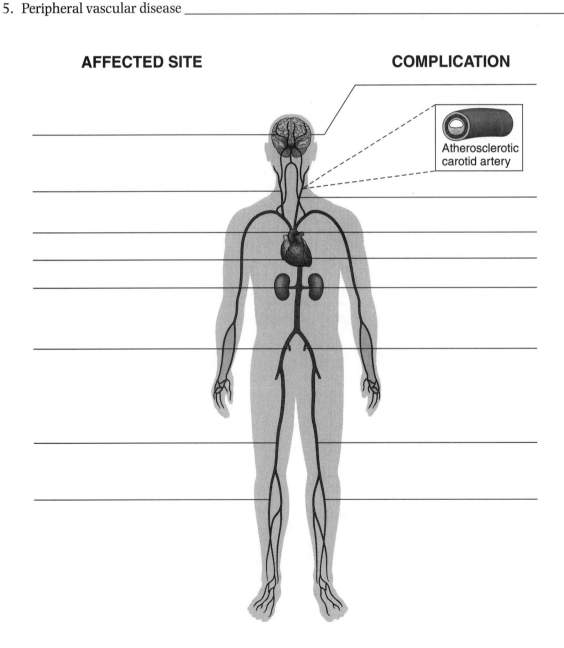

Atherosclerotic carotid artery

O. Complete the word puzzle relating to cerebral vascular accidents.

1. Acronym for condition   C __ __

2. May be affected in one eye   e __ __ __ __ __ __ __ __

3. Affected brain area causing
   left-sided hemiplegia   r __ __ __ __ __ __ __ __ __ __ __ __

4. A CAT scan is one of these   e __ __ __ __ __ __ __ __ __ __ __

5. Speech area of the brain   B __ __ __ __ ' __ __ __ __ __

6. General term for conditions that
   predispose people to CVA   r __ __ __ __ __ __ __ __ __ __

7. Result of immobility   a __ __ __ __ __ __ __

8. Affected brain area causing
   right-sided hemiplegia   l __ __ __ __ __ __ __ __ __ __

9. Dizziness   v __ __ __ __ __ __ __

10. Risk factor, vessel loses elasticity   a __ __ __ __ __ __ __ __ __ __ __ __ __ __ __

11. Another name for condition   s __ __ __ __ __ __

12. Common site where clots form   c __ __ __ __ __ __ __ __ __ __ __ __

13. Patient's complaint about limbs
    being affected   u __ __ __ __ __ __ __

14. Changes necessary to reduce risk of CVA   l __ __ __ __ __ __ __ __ __

15. Risk factor due to plaque buildup   a __ __ __ __ __ __ __ __ __ __ __ __ __ __

16. Treatments necessary to return to
    activities of daily living after CVA   r __ __ __ __ __ __ __ __ __ __ __ __ __ __

17. Loss of speech   a __ __ __ __ __ __ __

18. Diagnostic test used to assess
    cause of stroke   c __ __ __ __ __ __ __ __ __ __ __ __ __ __ __ __ __
    __ __ __ __ __ __ __ __ __

19. 90% of CVAs result from this   c __ __ __ __

20. When the brain is deprived of oxygen,
    this is the result   i __ __ __ __ __ __ __ __ __ __

21. Inability to say what one wants to   d __ __ __ __ __ __ __ __ __ __ in communicating

22. For treatment to be this, it must begin
    within 4 hours after stroke   e __ __ __ __ __ __ __ __ __ __

23. Test to determine reflexes after CVA   n __ __ __ __ __ - __ __ __ __ __

24. Where CVA places as a leading cause
    of death   t __ __ __ __ __

APPLYING THEORY TO PRACTICE

1. Prepare a presentation for junior high school students regarding nursing careers, including registered nurses, nurse clinicians, licensed practical nurses, and nurse aides. Describe the educational requirements, the role, and the future employment possibilities.

————————————————————————————————————

————————————————————————————————————

————————————————————————————————————

————————————————————————————————————

————————————————————————————————————

————————————————————————————————————

————————————————————————————————————

2. Why is hypertension called the "silent killer"?

————————————————————————————————————

————————————————————————————————————

3. What risk factors predispose people to hypertension?

————————————————————————————————————

————————————————————————————————————

4. What are the complications of hypertension?

————————————————————————————————————

————————————————————————————————————

5. How can hypertension be prevented?

————————————————————————————————————

SURF THE NET

Briefly summarize your findings from these Internet sites, or choose alternate sites for the following topics.

1. For information on the circulatory system, go to
   http://www.sirinet.net/~jgjohnso/circulation.html

2. Search for information on white coat hypertension. Report your findings.
   www.healthmonitor.com/TEMPRES/hart030598CS1.htm

3. For a fact sheet on stroke, go to http://www.caregiver.org/factsheets/strokeC.html

Lymphatic System and Immunity

OVERVIEW

The **lymphatic system** consists of the lymph, lymph nodes, vessels, spleen, thymus gland, tonsils, and lymphoid tissue in the intestinal tract.

Function of Lymph

Functions of the lymph system include the following:

Lymph fluid serves as the intermediary between blood in the capillaries and tissue.

Lymph vessels transport excess tissue fluid back into the circulatory system.

Lymph nodes produce lymphocytes and filter out harmful bacteria.

Spleen produces lymphocytes and monocytes, acts as a reservoir for blood, and recycles red blood cells.

Thymus gland produces T-lymphocytes.

Lymph is a straw-colored fluid similar to the blood plasma. **Intercellular** or **interstitial fluid** is lymph that bathes the spaces surrounding the tissue cells.

Lymph vessels accompany and closely parallel the venous system; they are located in almost all the tissues and organs that have blood vessels. They form two main ducts, the thoracic and right lymphatic.

Thoracic duct receives lymph from the left side of the chest, head, neck, abdominal area, and lower limbs and empties into the left subclavian vein.

Right lymphatic duct receives lymph from the right arm, right side of the head, and upper trunk and empties into the right subclavian vein.

Lymph nodes are oval structures located alone or grouped in places along the lymph vessels. They provide a site for lymphocyte production and serve as a filter for screening out harmful substances.

Tonsils are masses of lymph tissue, capable of producing lymphocytes and filtering out harmful bacteria. There are three pairs: the palatine, adenoids, and lingual.

The **spleen** is a saclike mass of lymphatic tissue located in the upper left area of the abdominal cavity. It forms lymphocytes and monocytes and stores and recycles large amounts of red blood cells.

The **thymus gland** is located in the thoracic area and produces T-lymphocytes and thymosin.

Effects of Aging

The immune system cells are no longer able to undergo rapid cell division that leaves every organ and tissue in the body more vulnerable to disease.

Disorders of the Lymph System

Lymphadenitis is the enlargement of the lymph nodes.

Hodgkin's disease is a form of cancer of the lymph nodes.

Infectious mononucleosis is caused by the Epstein-Barr virus spread by oral contact; also known as the kissing disease.

Immunity.   Immunity is the ability of the body to resist disease. There are two general types of immunity:

Natural is born with immunity.

Acquired is the result of exposure. Acquired immunity can be active or passive.

There are two types of *active acquired immunity:*

1. Natural—having the disease and recovering

2. Artificial—from a vaccination

There are also two types of *passive acquired immunity:*

1. Natural—may come from the mother's milk to the baby

2. Artificial—receiving serum from another (i.e., gamma globulin)

Immunization is the process of increasing an individual's resistance to a particular infection by artificial means.

Immunoglobulin is a protein that functions specifically as an antibody.

In **autoimmunity,** an individual's immune system forms antibodies against its own tissues causing autoimmune disorders, namely lupus and scleroderma.

Hypersensitivity occurs when the body's immune system fails to protect itself against foreign material; instead, antibodies formed irritate certain body cells.

Anaphylaxis or **anaphylactic shock** is a severe and sometimes fatal allergic reaction.

Acquired Immunodeficiency Syndrome (AIDS)

AIDS is caused by the human immunodeficiency virus (HIV), which suppresses the body's own immune system. The patient becomes susceptible to opportunistic infections that can normally be fought off by a healthy individual with a normally functioning immune system. The most common infections are Kaposi's sarcoma (blood vessel malignancy) and pneumocystic pneumonia.

Diagnostic Tests for AIDS.   Diagnostic tests include HIV antibody test, ELISA test, and Western blot test. Home-based test kits are available.

Symptoms of AIDS.   Symptoms of AIDS are nonspecific and are very similar to other illnesses, such as influenza.

The *incubation period* (the time between becoming infected and when the actual symptoms appear) is quite long, ranging from 1 month to 10 years.

AIDS-related complex (ARC) develops when an individual contracts the HIV, and symptoms occur; some individuals may develop AIDS.

Some people infected with HIV do not develop symptoms; this is called **asymptomatic infection.**

Treatment for AIDS.   Treatment for AIDS uses three classes of antiretroviral drugs.

High-Risk Groups for AIDS.   High-risk groups for AIDS include:

Homosexual and bisexual men with multiple sexual partners.

Male and female intravenous drug users who share needles.

Infants born to parents with AIDS.

Persons who received blood or blood products before all blood banks were required to test for HIV.

Transmission is by sexual intercourse, sharing of hypodermic needles, and infants born to parents who are HIV positive.

Measures to *prevent* transmission include limiting sexual partners, using latex condoms, and avoiding practices that would place people at risk of acquiring this disease.

ACTIVITIES

A.   Fill in the missing word or words.

1. The lymph system differs from the circulatory system because it lacks a

    _____.

2. Lymph fluid is the intermediary between the blood in the capillaries and the

    _____.

3. The spleen produces _____ and _____.

4. The spleen works as a recycling plant; the other organ with a similar function is the

    _____.

5. The transportation of excess fluid back into the circulatory system is accomplished by the

    _____.

6. The thymus gland is part of the lymph system and the _____

    _____.

7. Lymph nodes help in the defense of the body by filtering out _____

    _____.

8. The spleen helps the body in hemorrhagic conditions since it acts as a blood

    _____.

9. The organ of the lymph system located in the pharynx is the _____.

10. The type of white blood cell produced by the thymus gland is the _____.

B. Select the letter of the choice that best completes the statement.

1. Lymph is a straw-colored fluid that is also called:
   a. plasma
   b. serum
   c. interstitial
   d. intracellular

2. Lymph contains all of the following except:
   a. digested nutrients
   b. hormones
   c. granulocytes
   d. large protein molecules

3. The method by which lymph is pushed through the lymph vessels is:
   a. muscular pump
   b. contraction of the lymph vessels
   c. contraction of skeletal muscles against the lymph vessels
   d. contraction of smooth muscles against the lymph vessels

4. Lymph vessels closely resemble veins and may be found in the:
   a. central nervous system
   b. epidermis
   c. muscles
   d. spleen

5. Lymph in the thoracic duct area is carried to the:
   a. subclavian vein
   b. jugular vein
   c. brachial vein
   d. radial vein

6. Lymph travels in one direction:
   a. from the heart to body organs
   b. from body organs to pulmonary circulation
   c. from body organs to the heart
   d. from body organs to the liver

7. Swelling of the lymph tissue occurs because of an increase in:
   a. pathogenic substances
   b. white blood cells
   c. plasma fluid
   d. number of lymphocytes

8. Tonsils are masses of lymph tissue; the adenoid tonsils are located:
   a. under the tongue
   b. on the sides of the soft palate
   c. on the sides of the hard palate
   d. in the upper part of the throat

9. Enlargement of the tonsils causes all of the following except:
   a. difficulty in swallowing
   b. hoarseness
   c. sore throat
   d. pyrexia

10. As a person ages the size of the tonsils:
    a. does not change
    b. decreases slightly
    c. increases slightly
    d. decreases a lot

C. Label the diagram of lymph circulation. Color the red blood cells red and the lymph fluid yellow.

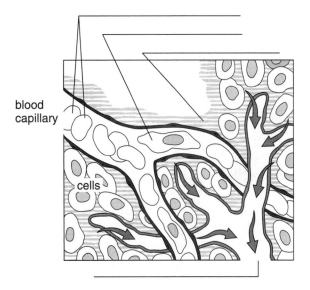

blood
capillary

cells

D. Compare the following items in terms of structure and function.

1. Blood capillary/lymph capillary

   _____

   _____

2. Thoracic duct/inferior vena cava

   _____

   _____

3. Intercellular fluid/intracellular fluid

   _____

   _____

4. Immunity/autoimmunity

E. Label the diagram of lymph drainage. Color the thoracic duct yellow, the right lymph duct blue, and the lymph nodes orange.

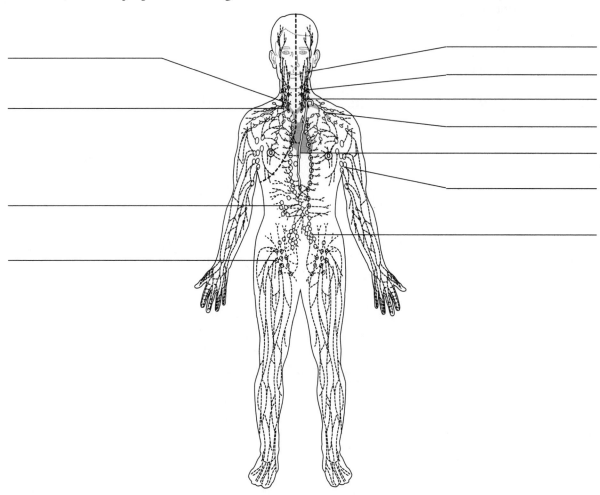

F. State each structure's location and function.

Structure	Location	Function
Spleen		
Thymus		
Axillary lymph node		
Thoracic duct		
Palatine tonsils		
Right lymph duct		
Lymph capillaries		

G. Fill in the blanks to complete the following statements.

1. Immunity is the ability to _____ disease.

2. Baby Anthony was born with anatomical barriers to disease; this is considered _____ immunity.

3. Rebecca, age 6, has had chickenpox and recovered; she now has _____ _____ immunity.

4. Kathy, working in the adult home center, has been exposed to hepatitis; she will receive an injection of gamma globulin, which will give her _____ _____ immunity.

5. Bryan is going to camp. The physical form asks whether he has received immunization to measles and mumps. This type of immunization is _____ _____ immunity.

6. Baby Megan's mother, Eileen, has had mumps, which will give Megan _____ _____ immunity; it will last only about 1 year.

H. The length of time immunity lasts varies; state the amount of time each type lasts.

1. Natural immunity   _____

2. Natural passive immunity   _____

3. Artificial acquired immunity   _____

4. Natural acquired immunity   _____

I. Circle the correctly spelled word in each of the following statements.

1. The term (swollen, swollan) glands is another term for lymph (adenitis, adanitis).

2. Treatments for Hodgkin's disease include chemotherapy and (radiation, rediation).

3. The lymph disease that often occurs in young adults and children is infectious (mononucleosis, mononuclosis).

4. Mono or the "kissing disease," is treated (symptomatically, symptomaticaly).

5. In autoimmunity, an (individual's, individeual's) immune system forms antibodies that attack healthy tissue.

6. In hypersensitivity reactions, the antibodies formed irritate certain body cells, causing an (alergic, allergic) reaction.

7. In asthma, antibodies bind to (bronchioles, broncholes); in hay fever they cause runny nose and (itcy, itchy) eyes.

8. A severe allergic reaction is called (anophylactic, anaphylactic) shock.

9. Patients should always be questioned regarding (sensativity, sensitivity) to allergens or drugs.

10. Medical-alert tags have saved the lives of people who are (unconsious, unconscious) or unable to communicate.

J. Answer the following questions about HIV and AIDS.

1. What do the HIV and AIDS acronyms mean?

_____

_____

2. Describe the earliest sign that a new disease is becoming prevalent.

_____

_____

3. Describe the similarities and differences of the following pairs.
   a. AIDS/ARC

   _____

   _____

   b. AIDS/asymptomatic infection

   _____

   _____

4. In the HIV antibody test, a positive result indicates what three things?

_____

_____

_____

5. What does a positive result in the ELISA test indicate?

_____

6. What does a positive Western blot test indicate?

_____

K. The following symptoms occur in AIDS patients. Name another condition in which these symptoms may also appear.

Symptom	Disorder
1. Prolonged fatigue	
2. Persistent cough	
3. Shortness of breath	
4. Chronic diarrhea	
5. Easy bruising or bleeding	
6. Discolored skin lesions	
7. Swollen glands	
8. Unexplained weight loss	

L. Define the following terms related to AIDS.

1. Opportunistic infection: _____

_____

2. Incubation period: _____

_____

3. Cytomegalovirus: _____

_____

4. AZT or similar antiretroviral drugs: _____

_____

5. Asymptomatic infection: _____

_____

M. Answer the following questions.

1. Name the four high-risk groups for AIDS.

_____

_____

2. List at least four situations in which a health care worker may be exposed to AIDS.

_____

_____

_____

_____

N. Place the following words in the crossword puzzle.

3 Letters
ARC
cut

4 Letters
AIDS
gown
mask
mono

5 Letters
cough
lymph
ulcer

6 Letters
gloves

plasma
spleen
thymus
valves

7 Letters
caution
dyspnea
goggles
lingual
natural
needles
passive
tonsils
vaccine

8 Letters
acquired
adenitis
adenoids
allergen
axillary
bleeding
Hodgkins
immunity
palatine

9 Letters
isolation
lymphatic

10 Letters
autoimmune
incubation
leukopenia
lymph nodes

11 Letters
anaphylaxis

12 Letters
immunization
interstitial
thoracic duct
transmission

13 Letters
opportunistic

14 Letters
Kaposis sarcoma

15 Letters
lymphatic
system
natural
acquired

16 Letters
acquired
immunity
hypersensitivity

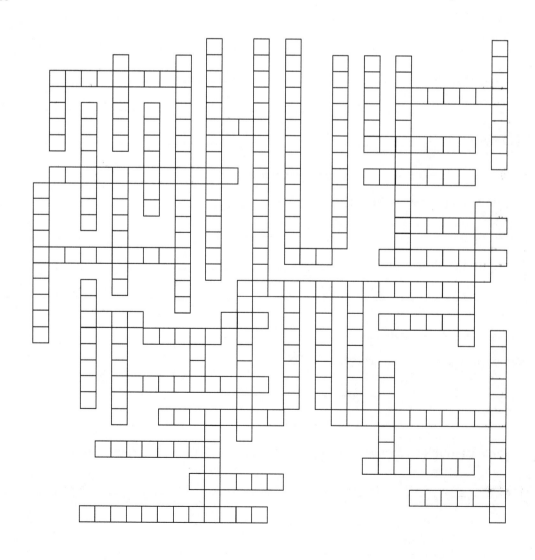

APPLYING THEORY TO PRACTICE

1. The patient's mother says that years ago if you had many sore throats the doctors would remove your tonsils. This procedure is not done for sore throats today. Why has the standard changed?

   _____

   _____

2. A father states that he does not want his baby vaccinated. How would you respond regarding immunization?

   _____

   _____

   _____

   _____

3. Meghan is a busy student who also works. She has been very tired over the past few weeks, is pale, and is experiencing some dyspnea. At the HMO she has blood tests done. The doctor, after examining the results of the blood tests, tells Meghan she has an autoimmune disease of the blood. What disease does Meghan have?

   _____

   _____

4. The residents in the nursing home are getting their annual flu shots. Mrs. Leona, an 80-year-old resident, says, "I had that before. Why do I need it again?" Explain to Mrs. Leona the reason for the flu shot.

   _____

   _____

5. As a medical assistant, what immunization is recommended and how is it administered?

   _____

   _____

6. Alan has an autoimmune disease of the skin. What skin disease other than scleroderma does Alan have?

   _____

   _____

7. Mike is a worker at an auto repair shop. He steps on a board there with nails. Mike goes to the ER for treatment. What questions will the paramedic have for Mike regarding immunization?

   _____

   _____

SURF THE NET

Briefly summarize your findings from the suggested Web sites, or choose alternate sites for the following topics.

1. For an immunization schedule for children, go to
   http://www.cdc.gov/mmwr/preview/mmwrhtml/mm5102a4.htm

2. For updates on autoimmune disease, go to
   http://www.niaid.nih.gov/publications/autoimmune/textonly.htm

3. For information about HIV/AIDS, go to http://www.ama-assn.org/special/hiv/hivhome.htm

Chapter 16

Infection Control
and Standard Precautions

OVERVIEW

Infection control principles that relate to pathogenic microorganisms include chain of infection, normal defense mechanisms, the infectious process, nosocomial infections, and standard precautions.

Flora

Flora are microorganisms that occur in a specific environment. There are two types of flora:

Resident flora or normal flora are always present.

Transient flora occur in periods of limited duration.

Pathogenicity and Virulence

Pathogenicity is the ability of microorganisms to produce disease. **Virulence** is the frequency with which a pathogen may cause disease.

Types of Microorganisms. The five types of pathogenic microorganisms are bacteria, virus, fungi, protozoa, and rickettsia.

Bacteria are one-celled microorganisms that lack a true nucleus or mechanism to provide metabolism; some types produce spores.

Virus is a microorganism that can only live inside a cell; some viruses produce a protective coat called an envelope.

Fungi may grow in single cells or colonies found mainly in people who are immunologically impaired.

Protozoa are single-celled organisms with the ability to move.

Rickettsia are intercellular parasites that need to be in living cells to reproduce. Infection is spread through the bite of fleas, ticks, and lice.

Chain of Infection

The **chain of infection** describes the elements of an infectious process. This process includes several essential elements for transmission of microorganisms to occur.

Agent.   An **agent** is an entity that is capable of causing disease, for example:

Biological agents are living organisms that invade the host such as bacteria, virus, fungi, protozoa, and rickettsia.

Chemical agents are substances that can interact with the body such as pesticides.

Physical agents are factors in the environment such as heat, light, noise, and radiation.

Reservoir.   The **reservoir** is a place where the agent can survive and reproduce. The most common reservoirs are humans, animals, environment, and **fomites** (objects contaminated with an infectious agent). **Carriers** are humans and animals that have the infectious agent but are symptom free.

Portal of Exit.   The **portal of exit** is the route by which an infectious agent leaves the reservoir through body secretions.

Mode of Transmission.   The **mode of transmission** is the process that bridges the gap between the portal of exit of the agent and the portal of entry of the susceptible new host. Types include the following:

Contact—physical transfer from an infected person to an uninfected person

Airborne—occurs when a susceptible person contacts contaminated droplets or dust particles suspended in the air

Vehicle—occurs when the agent is transferred to a susceptible host by contaminated inanimate objects such as water

Vectorborne—occurs when an agent is transferred to a susceptible person by mosquitoes, fleas, and ticks

Portal of Entry.   The **portal of entry** is the route by which an infectious agent enters the new host.

Host.   The **host** is an individual who is at risk of contracting an infection. A *susceptible host* is a person who lacks resistance and is vulnerable to disease. A *compromised host* is a person whose normal defense mechanisms are impaired and is more susceptible to infection.

Breaking the Chain of Infection

Health care workers focus on breaking the chain of infection by applying proper infection control practices to interfere with the spread of microorganisms.

Between Agent and Reservoir.   The key to eliminating infection is through cleansing, disinfection, and sterilization.

Between Reservoir and Portal of Exit.   Promoting proper hygiene, maintaining clean dressings and linen, and ensuring the use of clean equipment can break the chain.

Between Portal of Exit and Mode of Transmission. Maintaining clean dressings on all wounds, covering the mouth and nose when sneezing and coughing, using gloves with infectious secretions, and properly disposing of contaminated articles can break the chain.

Between Mode of Transmission and Portal of Entry. Break the chain by washing hands before and between patients and using barrier protection such as masks, gowns, gloves, and goggles.

Between Portal of Entry and Host. Maintain skin integrity and use sterile technique to prevent transmission from an infected person to an uninfected person.

Between Host and Agent. Proper nutrition, exercise, and immunization can maintain an intact immune system.

Normal Defense Mechanisms

The individual's immune system is a normal defense mechanism. A unique feature of the immune system is the ability to recognize antigens that are not consistent with the genetic makeup of the host.

Nonspecific Immune Defense. The nonspecific immune defense is not dependent on prior exposure to the antigen. Examples include the skin and normal flora; mucous membranes; sneezing, coughing, and tearing reflexes; elimination and acidic environment; and inflammation.

Specific Immune Defense. Specific immune defense is a response that is specific to the invading antigen and the production of T-lymphocyte cells (T-cells) and B-cells.

T-cells release substances called lymphokines that attract other lymphocytes to the area to assist in antigen destruction and stimulate production of B-cells.

B-cells cause formation of memory B-cells that remember the antigen and prepare the host for future antigen invasion.

Stages of the Infectious Process

The two types of infectious responses are *localized* (confined to one area) and *systemic* (affects the entire body). The stages are as follows:

Incubation—time interval between entry of an infection and the onset of symptoms

Prodromal—time interval from the onset of nonspecific symptoms until specific symptoms appear

Illness—time when the person is showing specific signs and symptoms

Convalescent—time from the beginning of disappearance of acute symptoms until the person returns to the previous state of health

Nosocomial Infections

A **nosocomial infection** is acquired in a hospital. Personnel who fail to follow proper handwashing techniques transmit most infections.

Standard Precautions

Standard precautions are the guidelines to be used during routine patient care and cleaning duties. They are required when there is possible contact with blood, any body fluid except sweat, mucous membranes, and nonintact skin. Standard precautions establish guidelines for handwashing, the use of protective barriers, care of patient equipment, occupational health, and bloodborne pathogens, as well as for patient placement.

ACTIVITIES

A. Complete the statement by filling in the correct answer.

1. Health care workers are responsible for care that utilizes _____ _____ principles to provide a safe environment.

2. Organisms that have the ability to live in a specific environment for a period of limited duration are known as _____ _____.

3. The ability of microorganisms to produce disease is known as _____.

4. _____ refers to the frequency with which a pathogen can cause disease.

5. An example of a resident flora is found on the _____.

B. Name the factors that affect the virulence of a pathogen.

_____

_____

_____

C. List the five types of pathogenic microorganisms.

_____

_____

_____

_____

_____

D. Select the letter of the choice that best completes the statement.

1. One-celled organisms that lack a true nucleus are:
   a. protozoa
   b. bacteria
   c. virus
   d. fungi

2. Malaria is a disease cause by:
   a. bacteria
   b. virus
   c. protozoa
   d. fungi

3. The ability to create an additional coating called an envelope is a characteristic of:
   a. virus
   b. bacteria
   c. protozoa
   d. rickettsia

4. Rocky Mountain spotted fever is caused by:
   a. virus
   b. bacteria
   c. protozoa
   d. rickettsia

5. A resistant state of bacterial production that can withstand unfavorable environments is known as:
   a. mold
   b. envelope
   c. spore
   d. parasite

6. Urinary tract infections are mostly caused by:
   a. rickettsia
   b. fungi
   c. virus
   d. bacteria

7. A single-celled organism that obtains food from dead or decaying organic matter is:
   a. protozoa
   b. virus
   c. fungi
   d. rickettsia

8. Measles are caused by a:
   a. protozoa
   b. virus
   c. fungi
   d. bacteria

9. An infection that is spread by the bites of fleas, ticks, and mites is a:
   a. fungal infection
   b. bacterial infection
   c. rickettsia infection
   d. protozoal infection

10. Individuals who are immunologically impaired may be more susceptible to disease caused by:
     a. virus
     b. fungi
     c. rickettsia
     d. bacteria

E.   Label the following diagram of the chain of infection.

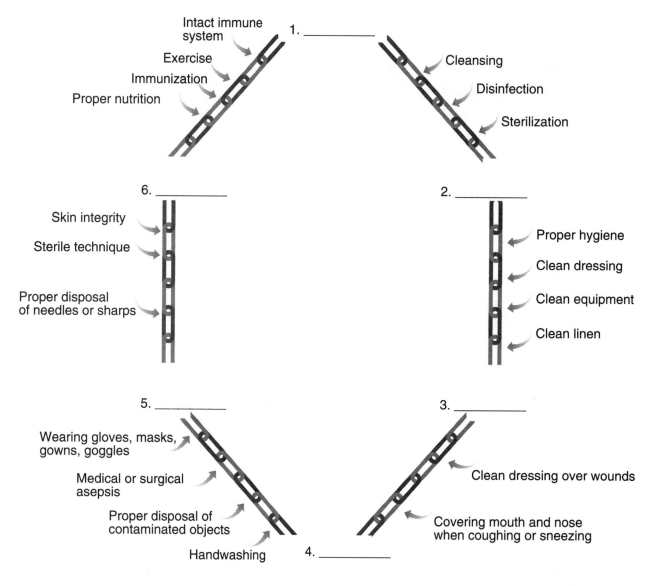

F.   Place the numbers from the previous diagram beside the best description.
     a. _____ Place where the agent can survive
     b. _____ A simple or complex organism that can be affected by an agent
     c. _____ Process that bridges the gap between portal of exit and portal of entry
     d. _____ An entity that is capable of causing disease
     e. _____ Route by which an infectious agent enters the host
     f. _____ Route by which an infectious agent leaves the host

G. Use information on practices that will break the chain of infection. Place your answer under the line for the rhyme.

> Example: A clean dressing goes over the wound
> Will help a person get well real soon
> <u>Between portal of entry and transmission</u>

1. Immunization, exercise, and good nutrition
   To keep healthy this is good ammunition

   _____

2. Disinfecting, sterilizing, and cleansing
   Will keep this pathogen from growing

   _____

3. Covering mouths when sneezing or coughing
   Will keep microbes from migrating

   _____

4. The pathogens cannot leave the scene
   If you use clean dressings and practice good hygiene

   _____

5. Wearing masks and gowns and washing hands
   Will keep germs from finding a new place to land

   _____

6. Skin integrity and sterile technique will help defeat
   These little microbes from finding a new place to eat

   _____

H. Mark the statement as either true or false. Correct the statement if false.

_____ 1. The skin and normal flora serve as physical agents against infectious agents.

_____ 2. Tears contain bactericides which inhibit bacterial growth.

_____ 3. The large intestines have an acidic environment to prevent growth of pathogens.

_____ 4. The nonspecific response to cell injury is inflammation.

_____ 5. The stimulation of T-cells and the production of antibodies are referred to as humoral immunity.

I. Compare the following terms.

1. Susceptible host and compromised host

   _____

2. T-cells and B-cells

   _____

3. Antigen and antibody

   _____

4. Direct contact transmission and indirect contact transmission

_____

5. Fomite and carrier

_____

J. Underline the correctly spelled word.

1. Localized and (systemic, systamic) infection progress through four stages.

2. An infection limited to a defined area is a (localized, localezed) infection.

3. The incubation stage is the time interval between entry of an infectious agent into the host and the onset of symptoms in the (infectous, infectious) process.

4. The time interval from the onset of nonspecific symptoms until specific symptoms appear occurs in the (prodomal, prodromal) stage of infection.

5. The period of time from the beginning of disappearance of acute symptoms until the patient returns to the previous state of health is the (convalescent, convalesent) stage.

6. A (nosocomial, nosocommial) infection is acquired in a hospital or other health care facility.

7. (Personnal, Personnel) who fail to follow proper handwashing techniques transmit most infections.

8. The hospital environment provides exposure to a (variety, variaty) of virulent organisms.

9. The most common endemic infection is a (urinery, urinary) tract infection.

10. Individuals in long-term care facilities have multiple illnesses which decrease their (resistence, resistance) to infection.

K. Handwashing is the single most effective way to prevent infection. Describe four rules that must be followed when handwashing.

_____

_____

_____

_____

L. When should a health care worker wear gloves?

_____

_____

_____

M. Describe how a health care worker can prevent injuries from needles.

_____

_____

_____

N. Word Search. Circle the key word related to infection control and standard precautions.

INFECTION CONTROL

```
n n f h f t n e c s e l a v n o c
f o o l o n o i t c e f n i s i d
w p s i o s a g n i s n a e l c f
y o s o t r t e n r o b r i a u b
y r t t c c a w q p t o u b n t m
t t e i r o e e k r y c k g n s v
i a r x i r m f x s h i i e i a i
c l i e o h w i n d i b g n x h r
i o l f v o l p a i w a a f u n u
n f i o r b v f j i f g v j q u l
e e z l e s g t v c r o s v v m e
g n a a s a r i a o e f n p h n n
o t t t e u r r o x e k o i o z c
h r i r r u r r b g h f i m a r e
t y o o s i c k w w z l i s i h e
a x n p e i p r o d r o m a l t c
p m v r m r i c k e t t s i a e e
```

agent
airborne
carrier
chain of infection
cleansing
convalescent
disinfection
flora
fomite
fungi
host
microorganism
nosocomial
pathogenicity
portal of entry
portal of exit
prodromal
reservoir
rickettsia
spore
sterilization
virulence
virus

APPLYING THEORY TO PRACTICE

1. Meghan, an LPN, works in a surgical ambulatory care setting. What are some of the infection control principles that Meghan must use in cleaning the equipment?

_____

_____

_____

_____

2. Vincent is the father of four children. He explains that colds in his household go from one person to another. Describe some of the methods of preventing colds from spreading in the household.

_____

_____

_____

_____

3. Since the September 11, 2001, attacks by terrorists, there is much fear in the public about bioterrorist attacks. Kreg works for a lumber supply company and asks Alyia, the nurse in the personnel department, what he should do in case of such a bioterrorist attack. What should Alyia tell Kreg?

_____

_____

_____

_____

4. Victoria is a visiting nurse for the Senior Center. Describe the characteristics she must be aware of that make a person more susceptible to infection.

_____

_____

_____

_____

5. Mike is an EMT. Under what circumstances should Mike wear barrier protection on the job?

_____

_____

_____

_____

SURF THE NET

Briefly summarize your findings from the suggested Web sites, or choose alternate sites for the following topics.

1. For immune system information, including nonspecific and specific immunity, go to, http://www.besthealth.com/bguide/bgready.html

2. Standard precautions from the CDC are at http://www.cdd.gov/ncidod/hip

3. Search for information on bioterrorism at http://www.bt.CDC.gov

Respiratory System

Chapter 17

OVERVIEW

The structures of the respiratory system allow for the exchange of oxygen and carbon dioxide for use by the cells of the body. This process is essential for the body to survive.

Functions of the Respiratory System. Functions of the respiratory system include the following:

To provide structures for the exchange of oxygen and carbon dioxide in the body and cells
To be responsible for the production of sound

Human respiration is divided into three stages:

External respiration is breathing or ventilation; exchange of CO_2 and O_2 occurs between the lungs and the outside environment.

Internal respiration is the exchange of O_2 and CO_2 between the cells and the lymph surrounding them.

Cellular respiration or *oxidation* is the use of oxygen to release energy stored in nutrient molecules. When food is oxidized, it gives off carbon dioxide and water as waste.

Organs of Respiration

Organs of respiration include the nasal cavity, sinuses, pharynx, larynx, trachea, bronchi, bronchioles, alveolar ducts, alveoli, lungs, pleura, and mediastinum.

Nasal Cavity. Air enters through the nasal cavity, which filters, moistens, and warms the air.

Anterior nares are two oval openings in the nose; also called the *nostrils.*
Nasal septum divides the nasal cavity into a right and left chamber.
Nasal concha or *turbinates* are three scroll-like bones that increase the surface area of the nasal cavity, causing turbulence.
Olfactory nerve is the upper part of the nasal cavity; it provides the sense of smell.

Sinuses. Sinuses are cavities lined with mucous membranes. They are located in the bones of the skull, around the nasal region, and are referred to as the *frontal, ethmoidal, maxillary,* and *sphenoidal* sinuses. They give tone to the voice.

Pharynx.   The pharynx, or throat, is the common passageway for food and air. Air goes from the nasal cavity to the pharynx, which is divided into three parts: the *nasopharynx*, *oropharynx*, and *laryngopharynx.*

Larnyx.   The larnyx, or voice box, is inferior to the pharynx. A cartilage lid, the *epiglottis*, is pushed by the tongue when you swallow to close the larynx, preventing food from entering the trachea. The larynx contains the *vocal cords;* air passes over the vocal cords to create sound.

Trachea.   The trachea, or windpipe, is a ciliated passageway that extends from the larynx to the bronchi. It is composed of 15 to 20 C-shaped cartilage rings.

Bronchi and Bronchioles.   The lower end of the trachea divides into the right and left bronchi. These bronchi further subdivide into smaller structures, the bronchioles. At the end of each bronchiole is an alveolar duct.

Alveolar Duct and Sacs.   At the end of each alveolar duct is the alveolar sac, which resembles a cluster of grapes and consists of many alveoli.

Alveoli.   The alveoli are a single layer of epithelial cells. The exchange of oxygen and carbon dioxide occurs between the capillaries around the alveoli by the process of diffusion. *Surfactant* is a lipid material that lines the inner surface of the alveoli.

Lungs.   The lungs are right and left cone-shaped organs in the thoracic cavity. Lung tissue is porous and spongy because of the tremendous amount of air it contains. The right lung is divided into three lobes, the left into two lobes.

Pleura.   The pleura is a double-layered membrane covering the lungs. The parietal pleura lines the thoracic cavity, and the visceral pleura covers the lung. Pleural fluid in this space prevents friction as the lungs expand and contract.

> *Pleurisy* is inflammation of the lining of the pleura.
> *Pneumothorax* is buildup of excess air in the pleural cavity on one side of the chest. The excess air increases pressure on the lung, causing it to collapse.

Mediastinum.   The mediastinum, or interpleural space, is located between the lungs and extends from the sternum to the vertebrae.

Mechanics of Breathing (Ventilation)

Breathing Process.   Pulmonary ventilation allows the exchange of oxygen between the alveoli and the red blood cells.

> *Inhalation* or *inspiration* occurs when muscles in the thoracic cavity contract, increasing the space within the chest cavity. This results in a decrease in pressure; atmospheric pressure is now greater and air rushes in, all the way down to the alveoli.
> *Exhalation* or *expiration* is the opposite of inhalation. The muscles relax, space in the thoracic cavity decreases, and the increased pressure forces air out of the lungs.

Respiratory Movements. An inspiration and an expiration are one respiratory movement; the average rate is 14 to 20 breaths per minute. Factors that affect the rate are exercise, temperature, age, body position, emotions, coughing, sneezing, and hiccoughing.

Control of Breathing. The rate of breathing is controlled by neural and chemical factors.

Neural factors are controlled by the medulla oblongata in the brain. There are two centers, inspiratory and expiratory. An increase of carbon dioxide and a decrease of oxygen will trigger the respiratory center.

Phrenic nerves stimulate the diaphragm and the intercostal muscles.

Vagus nerves are involved in the Hering-Breuer reflex: when the lungs are inflated, the nerve endings of the lungs are stimulated, which then stimulate the vagus nerve to inhibit the inspiratory center.

Chemical factors occur as the level of carbon dioxide in the blood passes through the brain, stimulating the inspiration center.

Chemoreceptors are chemical regulators in the carotid arteries and aorta sensitive to the oxygen level; as oxygen decreases, impulses are sent to the respiratory center to stimulate inspiration.

Lung Capacity and Volume. Terms used to determine the amount of air in the lungs include *tidal volume, inspiratory reserve volume (IRV), expiratory reserve volume (ERV), vital capacity, residual volume, functional residual,* and *total lung capacity.* See Figure 17-9 in your textbook for further explanation of these terms.

Types of Respiration

The following terms relate to types of respiration.

Apnea: temporary stoppage of respiration

Dyspnea: difficulty in respiration

Eupnea: normal or easy breathing

Hyperpnea: increase in the depth and rate of breathing

Orthopnea: difficult or labored breathing in the horizontal position

Tachypnea: abnormally rapid and shallow breathing

Hyperventilation: condition caused by stress—rapid breathing causes a rapid loss of carbon dioxide, leading to alkalosis, which results in dizziness and fainting

Effects of Aging

The lung tissue loses elasticity and muscle strength decreases. These factors compromise oxygen and carbon dioxide exchange which causes signs of activity intolerance. There is a change in lung capacity. The elderly are more prone to respiratory disease.

Disorders of the Respiratory System

The *common cold* is the most common respiratory infection caused by a virus; it is often the basis for more serious disorders.

Infectious Causes.   Infectious causes include:

  Pharyngitis: red, inflamed throat

  Laryngitis: inflammation of the larynx or voice box

  Sinusitis: infection of the mucous membrane lining the sinuses

  Bronchitis: inflammation of the mucous membrane lining of the bronchial tubes; may be acute or chronic

  Influenza or *"flu":* inflammation of the respiratory system

  Pneumonia: infection of the lungs caused by a virus or bacteria

  Tuberculosis: disease of the lungs caused by the tubercle bacillus

  Diphtheria and *pertussis:* whooping cough; rarely seen today because children are immunized against these conditions shortly after birth.

  Anthrax: (inhalation) caused by the bacterium bacillus and its spores; spores convert to active bacillus and infect the lungs, leading to death

Noninfectious Causes.   Noninfectious causes include:

  Nasal polyps: growths in the sinus cavity that cause obstruction of the airway

  Rhinitis: inflammation of the nasal mucous membrane caused by an allergen or cold virus

  Asthma: airway becomes obstructed due to an inflammatory response to a stimulus that may be an allergen or stress

  Atelectasis: failure of lungs to expand normally due to bronchial occlusion

  Bronchiectasis: dilation of a bronchus caused by an inflammation

  Asbestosis: caused by inhaling asbestos fibers

  Silicosis: caused by breathing dust containing silicon dioxide; the lungs become fibrosed, which results in reduced lung capacity

  Pulmonary embolism: a blood clot that travels to the lung; may occur after a person has been immobile for a while.

Chronic Obstructive Pulmonary Disease (COPD).

  Emphysema is when the alveoli become overdilated, lose their elasticity, cannot rebound, and eventually rupture. In this process, air becomes trapped, making it difficult to exhale.

  Chronic bronchitis is also classified as COPD.

Cancers of the Respiratory System.

  Cancer of the lung is a malignant tumor that forms in the bronchial epithelium; the most common cause of lung cancer is smoking.

  Cancer of the larynx is a malignant tumor of the voice box.

Sudden Infant Death Syndrome (SIDS).   Sudden infant death syndrome, or *crib death,* usually occurs between the ages of 1 week and 1 year; the infant stops breathing during sleep, exact cause is unknown.

ACTIVITIES

A. Select the word or words from the following list to complete the statements. Word or words may be used more than once.

alveoli	diffuses	internal respiration
bicarbonate	exhalation	oxidation
breathing	external respiration	oxygen
carbon dioxide	inhalation	water
cellular respiration	inspiration	

1. The exchange of oxygen and carbon dioxide between the lungs and the environment is called _____ _____ or _____.

2. The ventilation process consists of taking air in, _____ and breathing air out, _____.

3. In ventilation, oxygen _____ from an area of higher concentration in the alveoli to an area of lower concentration in the bloodstream.

4. In the process of exhalation, _____ _____ and _____ are exhaled.

5. The exchange of carbon dioxide and oxygen between the cells and the surrounding lymph is called _____ _____.

6. Deoxygenated blood produced during internal respiration carries carbon dioxide in the form of _____ ions.

7. The use of _____ to release energy stored in nutrient molecules is called _____ _____ or _____.

8. The waste products of oxidation are carried away through the process of _____ _____.

B. Describe the functions of the respiratory system.

_____

_____

_____

_____

C. Label the diagram of the respiratory system. Trace air from the external environment to the alveoli. Color the diagram.

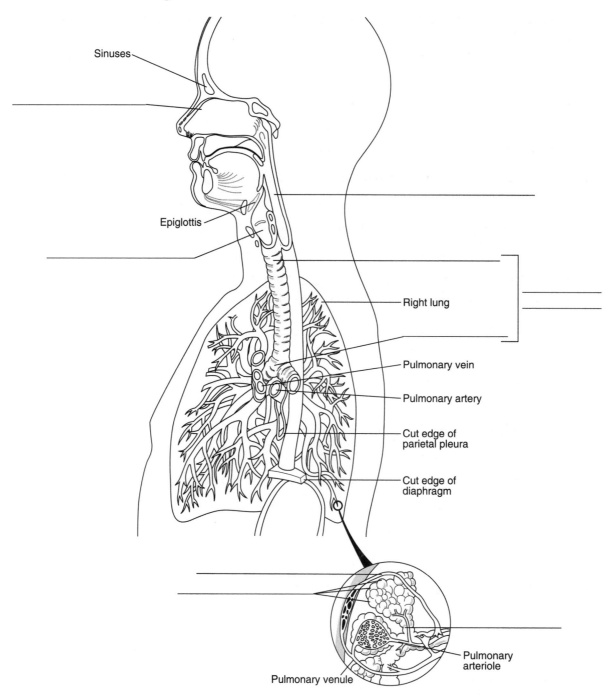

Sinuses

Epiglottis

Right lung

Pulmonary vein

Pulmonary artery

Cut edge of parietal pleura

Cut edge of diaphragm

Pulmonary arteriole

Pulmonary venule

D. Select the letter of the choice that best completes the statement.

1. The nasal cavities are lined with mucous membrane, and the:
   a. air is warmed and moistened as it goes through
   b. air is cooled and moistened as it goes through
   c. air is warmed and dried as it goes through
   d. air is cooled and dried as it goes through

2. The turbinates, or nasal concha, are responsible for:
   a. cooling the air in the nares
   b. filtering the air in the nasal cavity
   c. decreasing the surface area of the nasal cavity, causing turbulence
   d. increasing the surface area of the nasal cavity, causing turbulence

3. The structure that filters the air in the nasal cavity is the:
   a. concha
   b. cilia
   c. septum
   d. mucous membrane

4. Located in the upper part of the nasal cavity are the endings of the:
   a. otic nerve
   b. olfactory nerve
   c. oculomotor nerve
   d. auditory nerve

5. Air is warmed and moistened by all of the following structures except the:
   a. mucous membranes of the sinuses
   b. blood vessels
   c. mucous membrane
   d. cilia

6. The four nasal sinuses are the:
   a. frontal, ethmoidal, sphenoidal, and maxillary
   b. frontal, ethmoidal, sphenoidal, and mandible
   c. frontal, parietal, sphenoidal, and maxillary
   d. frontal, ethmoidal, sphenoidal, and temporal

7. The pharynx is also known as the:
   a. voice box
   b. windpipe
   c. throat
   d. nares

8. The eustachian tube connects the middle ear and the:
   a. laryngopharynx
   b. larynx
   c. nasopharynx
   d. propharynx

9. The opening to the larynx is closed when a cartilage lid called the epiglottis is pushed by the:
   a. propharynx
   b. nasopharynx
   c. mucous membrane of the nasal cavity
   d. tongue

10. Sound is produced when the air is:
    a. inhaled into the lungs
    b. exhaled from the lungs
    c. vibrated by the glottis
    d. acted on by the lips and tongue

E. The various sinuses are shown in the following diagram.

1. Label the sinuses.

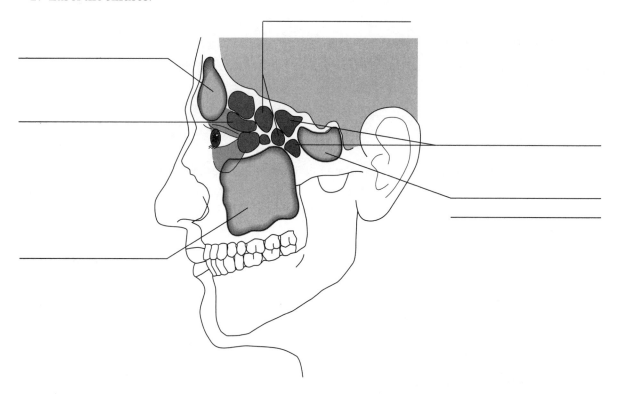

2. Describe the locations and functions of the sinuses.

_____

_____

_____

_____

F. Fill in the blanks to complete the statements on the respiratory system.

1. The trachea conducts air from the larynx to the _____ or

   _____ _____.

2. The walls of the trachea are composed of 15 to 20 C-shaped rings of _____

   _____, which prevent the trachea from collapsing.

3. The process by which dust-laden mucus is expelled is _____.

4. The lower end of the trachea divides into the _____ _____ and the _____ .

5. The terminal ends of the bronchi are the _____ .

6. The bronchiole walls are made from _____ _____ and elastic tissue lined with _____ epithelium.

7. At the end of the bronchiole there is an alveolar duct, which ends in a _____ _____ .

8. There are about _____ times the number of alveoli necessary to sustain life.

9. The inner surfaces of the alveoli are covered with _____ .

10. It is through the moist walls of the _____ and the _____ that rapid exchange of carbon dioxide and oxygen occurs.

G. Compare the following pairs according to structure and function.

1. Right bronchus/left bronchus

_____

_____

2. Lining of the trachea/lining of the bronchi

_____

_____

3. Alveolar duct/alveoli

_____

_____

4. Parietal pleura/visceral pleura

_____

_____

5. Right lung/left lung

_____

_____

6. Lung tissue/heart tissue

_____

_____

7. Pleurisy/pneumothorax

_____

_____

H. Use the words from the following list to complete the statements.

atmospheric pressure	elasticity	inspiration
compliance	expanded	internal intercostals
decrease	external intercostals	negative pressure
diaphragm	flattened	surface tension
downward	increases	upward

1. The normal pressure within the pleural space is always _____ _____, which is less than _____ _____; this helps keep the lungs expanded.

2. There are two groups of intercostal muscles; during _____, the _____ _____ lift the ribs _____ and outward.

3. During inspiration, the _____ contracts and becomes _____.

4. The action of the muscles and the diaphragm results in a _____ in pressure in the pleural space; the atmospheric pressure is greater and air rushes in.

5. In expiration, the _____ _____ of the fluid lining the alveoli reduces the elasticity of the lung tissue, causing the alveoli to collapse.

6. The ability of the lungs to change capacity as the size of the thoracic cavity is altered is known as _____.

I. Answer the following questions on respiration.

1. What actions are considered as one respiratory movement?

_____

2. What is the normal respiratory rate?

_____

3. How is the respiratory rate affected by the following?
    a. Age _____
    b. Body position _____
    c. Increased body temperature _____
    d. Gender _____
    e. Emotions _____

4. Explain how coughing, sneezing, and hiccoughing affect respirations.

_____

_____

_____

J. Breathing is controlled by neural factors and chemical factors. Explain the role of the following in respiratory control.

1. Medulla oblongata

_____

_____

2. Phrenic nerve

_____

_____

3. Vagus nerve

_____

_____

4. Hering-Breuer reflex

_____

_____

5. Increase in carbon dioxide

_____

_____

6. Chemoreceptor

_____

_____

7. Depressant drugs

_____

_____

K. Match the terms in Column A with the statements in Column B.

Column A	Column B
_____ 1. spirometer	a. includes tidal volume, IRV, ERV, and residual air
_____ 2. tidal volume	b. the total amount of air involved with tidal volume, IRV, and ERV
_____ 3. inspiratory reserve volume	c. air that cannot be voluntarily expelled from the lungs
_____ 4. expiratory reserve volume	d. amount of air that moves in and out of the lungs with one breath
_____ 5. total lung capacity	e. amount of air you can force a person to take in
_____ 6. residual volume	f. instrument that measures lung capacity
_____ 7. functional residual volume	g. amount of air you can force a person to exhale
	h. sum of the ERV plus the residual volume

L. Label the diagram of lung capacity and include the amount of air involved.

TOTAL LUNG CAPACITY (6,000 ml or 6L)

_____ → 500 ml

_____ 3000 ml ⎫ 4500 ml

Expiratory reserve volume (ERV) _____ ml

_____ 2500 ml

Residual air _____ → 1500 ml

M. Define the following terms.

1. Apnea: _____

_____

2. Dyspnea: _____

_____

3. Eupnea: _____

_____

4. Hyperpnea: _____

_____

5. Orthopnea: _____

_____

6. Tachypnea: _____

_____

7. Hyperventilation: _____

_____

N. How do you correct hyperventilation?

_____

_____

_____

_____

O. Use the words from the following list to complete the rhymes.

alveolar duct	bronchus	larynx	trachea
alveoli	capillary	mucus	vein
artery	cilia	nasal cavity	voice box
bronchi	inhaled	pharynx	

I was floating by in the evening breeze
when I got inhaled by a great big sneeze.

Next thing I knew I was inhaled inside
to the _____ _____ on the right side.

The place was warm, moist, and had _____ so thick
with little hairs called _____, they make you want to itch.

I did not have much chance to look around;
I went over the cliff and down, down, down.

I landed in a place called the _____ or throat;
it was so full of watery juice, I thought I needed a boat.

I was quickly pulled through a place with a high pitch,
the _____ or voice box where air rushes by real quick.

Off to another tube, lined with those little hairs;
windpipe or _____, I spent little time there.

I landed then on what looked like a tree;
the _____ I believe, what side should it be?

The _____ branches keep getting narrower and end in the _____
_____, into the air sacs or _____ I quickly get sucked.

I pass through the wall onto the _____ train;
off to a new adventure as I board an _____ and not a _____.

P. Circle the correctly spelled word in each of the following statements.

1. The common cold, a (resperatory, respiratory) infection, results in the greatest loss in production hours each year.

2. To treat a common cold you should stay in bed, drink plenty of fluid, and eat (wholesome, holesome), nourishing food.

3. (Pharyngitis, pharynxitis) is an inflammation of the throat that may occur as the result of an (irritant, irritent) such as too much smoking or speaking.

4. The most common form of laryngitis is (catarrhal, catarhal).

5. Symptoms of laryngitis include dryness, hoarseness, coughing, and (disphagia, dysphagia).

6. Sinusitis is an infection of the mucous membrane lining the sinus cavity or (cavities, cavites).

7. Acute bronchitis is characterized by fever, cough, substernal pain, and (rails, rales).

8. Chronic bronchitis differs from acute bronchitis in that the cough must be (persistent, persistence) for 3 months and have occurred for 2 consecutive years.

9. In (neumonia, pneumonia) an infection of the lung, the alveoli become filled with thick fluid called exudate.

10. An inflammation of the mucous membrane of the respiratory system is called the flu or (influenza, influinza).

Q. Answer the following questions.

1. Define tuberculosis.

   _____

   _____

2. What organs may be affected by tuberculosis?

   _____

   _____

3. In pulmonary tuberculosis, lesions called _____ form within the lung tissue.

4. Name the classic symptoms of tuberculosis.

   _____

   _____

5. The diagnostic test for TB is the _____ test, which is a skin test. It is read

   within _____ to _____ hours after the test.

6. Describe the treatment for tuberculosis.

   _____

   _____

   _____

7. These other two respiratory diseases are rarely seen today because children receive

   immunization against _____ and _____.

R. Match the following respiratory disorders in column A with the statements in column B
describing them.

Column A	Column B
_____ 1. nasal polyps	a. lungs fail to expand normally
_____ 2. rhinitis	b. dilatation of the bronchus accompanied by heavy pus secretions
_____ 3. asthma	c. lungs become fibrosed, leading to reduced capacity
_____ 4. atelectasis	d. inflammation of the nasal mucous membrane
_____ 5. bronchiectasis	e. growth that occurs in the nasal cavity
_____ 6. silicosis	f. airway obstructed due to an inflammatory response to a stimulus

S. Answer the following questions about lung disorders.

1. Name two conditions that are considered chronic obstructive pulmonary disease.

   _____

   _____

2. Describe what occurs to the alveoli of the lungs in emphysema.

   _____

   _____

3. Describe a surgical procedure that will help patients with emphysema.

   _____

T. Fill in the blanks to complete the following statements about lung cancer.

1. Cancer of the lungs is found mainly in people who _____.

2. Diagnosis of cancer of the lung is made usually by a _____. During this
   procedure, the throat is anesthetized; therefore it is important to be certain that the
   _____ _____ has returned before the person takes fluid
   or food.

APPLYING THEORY TO PRACTICE

1. In the drug store you find many preparations to treat colds. Compare at least five preparations, looking at factors such as ingredients, dosage, number of tablets in bottle, and cost. What did you learn to help you make better choices when you need a cold preparation?

2. What is the difference between a cough expectorant and a cough suppressant? Which respiratory structures are affected by each?

3. What produces sound and speech?

4. A patient who has been in bed recovering from hip surgery complains of sudden severe chest pain and is having dyspnea. What could be occurring?

5. The Jones family is very upset. They feel responsible for their infant's death from sudden infant death syndrome. Explain to the Jones family what you know about this condition.

6. Kayla's parents say she is having a great deal of difficulty in breathing. Kayla, age 5, has been previously treated in the ER for asthma. What are the causes of asthma; describe the physiological changes that occur in an asthmatic attack. Describe the usual treatment and a possible adjunct treatment for asthma? How can the nurse help Kayla understand her illness?

_____

_____

_____

7. Many people worry today about a terrorist attack. Why is there such fear regarding an anthrax attack?

_____

_____

_____

8. Maria is 78 years old; she has been very active at the Senior Center and loves to dance. Lately, Maria is having some difficulty in breathing after her dancing. As the LPN who is assigned to the Senior Center, explain to Maria what is occurring as she ages.

_____

_____

_____

SURF THE NET

Briefly summarize your findings from the suggested Web sites, or choose alternate sites for the following topics.

1. For structure and function information of the respiratory system, go to
   http://www.lungusa.org/learn/resp_sys.html

2. To take a quiz on the respiratory system, go to
   http://www.sk.lung.ca/education/student/games/swin.html

3. To learn more about types of respiration, go to http://www.e-respiration.net.

4. For additional facts on anthrax, go to
   http://www.cdc.gov/ncidod/dbmd/diseaseinfo/anthrax_g.htm

Digestive System

The organs of digestion change food into a simple form that can be used by the cells of the body and eliminate the waste products of the digestive process.

Digestion. Digestion is the process of changing complex solid foods into simple soluble forms that can be absorbed by the body cells.

The **digestive system** consists of the main organs of digestion: mouth, pharynx, esophagus, stomach, small intestine, large intestine, and anus. The accessory organs of digestion are the tongue, teeth, salivary glands, pancreas, liver, and gallbladder.

Layers of the Digestive System. The digestive system is composed of four layers:

Mucosa: the innermost lining, made of epithelial cells
Submucosa: connective tissue
Circular muscle: third layer
Longitudinal muscle: fourth layer

Lining of the Digestive System. The **peritoneum** is a serous double membrane lining the abdominal cavity. Specialized layers are as follows:

Mesentery: intestines attached to the lining, which is attached to the posterior wall of the abdominal cavity
Greater omentum: double fold of peritoneum that hangs down over the abdominal organs like an apron

Main Organs of Digestion

Mouth or Buccal Cavity. The mouth is the oral cavity. It is composed of several parts:

Hard palate: roof of the mouth, formed from maxillary and palatine bones
Soft palate: made from a movable mucous fold; separates the mouth from the nasopharynx
Uvula: conical flap that hangs from the soft palate

Tongue (Accessory Organ). The tongue is a bundle of skeletal muscles lying in many different planes.

> *Papillae* are projections of the tongue containing the nerve endings for taste buds.
>
> *Taste buds* are organs that sense salt, bitter, sour, and sweet flavors.

Salivary Glands (Accessory Organ). The three salivary glands, parotid, sublingual, and submandible, are located in the mouth; they produce a watery substance called saliva. Saliva softens and lubricates food and dissolves it. Saliva contains ptyalin (salivary amylase), which digests starch to simpler substances.

Teeth (Accessory Organ). Teeth cut and shred food, a process called mastication.

> **Gingivae,** or **gums,** are fleshy tissue, covered with mucous membrane, that support and protect the teeth. **Deciduous teeth** or **baby teeth** begin to erupt at 6 months and continue to 2 years of age. **Permanent teeth** begin to replace deciduous teeth at about 5 years; the adult mouth has 32 permanent teeth. Types of teeth are:

> *Incisors:* sharp edges for biting
>
> *Canines:* pointed for tearing
>
> *Molars:* ridges or cusps designed for crushing and grinding
>
> *Bicuspids:* premolars that are broad and have two cusps

Esophagus. The esophagus is a muscular tube about 10 inches long. It begins at the pharynx or throat and runs to the cardiac sphincter of the stomach.

Stomach. The stomach lies in the upper quadrant of the abdominal cavity and is divided into the *fundus, body,* and *pylorus.* When the stomach is empty, it hangs in folds called *rugae.* The opening between the esophagus and the stomach is controlled by the *cardiac sphincter;* the opening between the pylorus and the duodenum is controlled by the *pyloric sphincter.*

Gastric Glands. The gastric glands are located in the mucosal lining; they secrete pepsinogen, mucus, hydrochloric acid, and the intrinsic factor.

> *Pepsinogen* converts to pepsin by the action of hydrochloric acid.
>
> *Mucus* neutralizes the effects of hydrochloric acid.
>
> *Hydrochloric acid* destroys bacteria in food.
>
> *Intrinsic factor* is necessary for vitamin B_{12} absorption.

Small Intestine. The small intestine is a coiled portion of the digestive system about 20 feet long and 1 inch in diameter. It is divided into the duodenum (first 12 inches), the jejunum (8 feet), and the ileum (10 to 12 feet). A few inches into the duodenum is the ampulla of Vater, the site where the pancreatic duct and the common bile duct empty their contents into the small intestine. The digestive juices in the small intestine are the following:

> *Secretin and cholecystokinin* are enzymes that stimulate the digestive juices of the pancreas, liver, and gallbladder.
>
> *Pancreatic juices* break down protein, starch, and fats; they also contain sodium bicarbonate, which neutralizes the food content of the stomach.
>
> *Bile* emulsifies fat.
>
> *Intestinal juices* work on protein, starches, and fats.

Absorption in the Small Intestine.   Absorption in the small intestine is possible because of the *villi,* which contain blood capillaries and lymph capillaries that absorb the end products of digestion, including:

> *Starch:* absorbed as glucose
> *Protein:* absorbed as amino acids
> *Fat:* absorbed as fatty acids and glycerol

> See Table 18-1 of your textbook for additional information.

Accessory Organs of Digestion

The accessory organs of digestion are the tongue, teeth, salivary glands, pancreas, liver, and gallbladder.

Pancreas.   A feather-shaped organ behind the stomach, the pancreas produces digestive juices, insulin, and glucagon.

Liver.   The liver is located in the upper right quadrant and is the largest organ in the body. Its functions include:

> Manufacturing bile
> Manufacturing plasma proteins
> Detoxifying drugs and alcohol
> Storing glucose in the form of glycogen and storing Vitamins A, D, and B complex
> Preparing urea
> Breaking down hormones
> Removing worn out RBCs and recycling the iron content

Gallbladder.   The gallbladder is a small organ on the inferior surface of the liver. It stores and concentrates bile.

Large Intestine.   The large intestine or *colon* is about 5 feet long and 2 inches in diameter and includes the following:

> *Ileocecal valve:* connects the ileum to the colon.
> *Cecum:* blind pouch below the ileocecal valve; projecting from it is the vermiform appendix.

> The **colon** is divided into *ascending, transverse,* and *descending* parts. The large intestine absorbs water and contains normal flora that synthesize B-complex vitamins and vitamin K.
> The **sigmoid** portion is the end portion of the colon; it enters the iliac region and continues as the rectum.
> The **rectum** opens exteriorly to the anus, which contains the internal (involuntary) and the external (voluntary) muscle sphincters.
> **Defecation** is the reflex triggered when the rectum becomes distended, resulting in emptying of the bowels.

General Overview of Digestion

Food enters the mouth and is mechanically broken up by the teeth and chemically digested by saliva, at which point the food is called a *bolus.* The bolus moves into the pharynx and slides down to the esophagus, stomach, and small intestine where the food becomes totally fluid and is transported across the small intestine villi to the bloodstream. Undigested food goes to the large intestine and leaves through the anus as feces. Food is pushed through the system by peristalsis and segmented movement.

Action in the Organs.   The following organs are involved in digestion.

Mouth: teeth and tongue begin mechanical digestion by breaking food apart.

Salivary glands: in the mouth, the glands begin chemical digestion as ptyalin begins to change starch to maltose or glucose.

Pharynx: swallowing.

Esophagus: peristalsis and gravity move food into the stomach.

Stomach: hydrochloric acid prepares the area for action. Pepsin breaks up protein, and lipase acts on emulsified fats. Food leaves as chyme.

Liver: produces bile.

Gallbladder: stores and releases bile as needed.

Pancreas: enzymes are released into the small intestine: amylase breaks down starch, protease breaks down protein, and steapsin breaks down fat.

Small intestine: produces enzymes, prepares food for absorption, breaking it into glucose, amino acids, fatty acids, and glycerol; site for absorption.

Large intestine: absorbs water and collects food residue for excretion.

Effect of Aging

There is a decrease in the sensory ability of the taste buds and production of saliva. There may be a loss of teeth, which leads to poor nutrition. A slowdown in peristalsis may make it more difficult to swallow, digest food, and eliminate waste products.

Common Disorders of the Digestive System

Following are the common disorders of the digestive system.

Stomatitis is inflammation of the soft tissue of the mouth.

Gastroesophageal reflux (GERD) occurs when the cardiac sphincter muscle relaxes, and food flows back into the esophagus.

Hiatal hernia occurs when stomach tissue protrudes above the diaphragm through the esophageal opening.

Heartburn is backflow of acidic gastric juice into the lower end of the esophagus.

Pyloric stenosis is the narrowing of the pyloric sphincter.

Gastritis is inflammation of the lining of the stomach.

Gastroenteritis is inflammation of the lining of the stomach and intestines.

Enteritis is inflammation of the lining of the small intestine.

Peptic ulcers are lesions that occur in the stomach or duodenum; common cause is bacteria, *H. pylori.*

Appendicitis is inflammation of the vermiform appendix.

Hepatitis is inflammation of the liver. Types are:

Hepatitis A, viral hepatitis: spread through contaminated food and water.

Hepatitis B, serum hepatitis: caused by a virus found only in the blood.

Hepatitis C is caused by hepatitis virus, steadily growing disease hepatitis D, and hepatitis E.

Standard precautions are required for all types of hepatitis.

Cirrhosis is a chronic progressive disease of the liver; normal tissue is replaced by fibrous connective tissue.

Cholecystitis is inflammation of the gallbladder.

Gallstones are a collection of crystallized cholesterol that may block the bile duct.

Pancreatitis is inflammation of the pancreas.

Diverticulosis occurs when little sacs form in the intestine; if they become inflamed, diverticulitis develops.

Diarrhea is loose, watery, frequent bowel movements.

Constipation is when defecation is delayed; the colon absorbs excessive water from the feces, rendering them dry and hard; defecation thus becomes difficult.

Cancer may occur in any part of the digestive system. Surgery, chemotherapy, and radiation are available treatments.

Irritable Bowel Syndrome (IBD) is an inflammation of the intestinal tract; the most frustrating symptom is chronic diarrhea. The two types are: (1) Crohn's disease; inflammation occurs anywhere in the digestive tract and, (2) ulcerative colitis; inflammation typically occurs in the colon and rectum.

ACTIVITIES

A. Use the words in the following list to complete the statements.

alimentary canal	30 feet	mucosa
colon	gullet	pancreas
circular muscle	greater omentum	peritoneum
digestion	mesentery	small intestine
15 feet	insoluble complex	submucosa

1. To change food into simpler soluble molecules, physical and chemical changes occur; this process is known as _____.

2. The gastrointestinal tract is also known as the _____ _____.

3. Another name for the food tube or esophagus is the _____.

4. Muscle tone reduces the length of the alimentary canal to _____.

5. The first layer of the digestive tract insulates it from powerful enzymes and secretes digestive juices. It is known as the _____.

6. The third layer of the digestive system consists of _____ _____.

7. An accessory organ of digestion is the _____.

8. Lining the abdominal cavity is the _____ membrane.

9. A specialized layer of the membrane to which the small intestine is attached, and that is attached to the posterior wall of the abdominal cavity, is the _____.

10. This layer of the membrane hangs over the organs like a protective apron; it is known as the

_____ _____.

B. Answer the following questions regarding the digestive system.

1. Name the functions of the digestive system.

_____

_____

_____

_____

2. Why are some of the organs called accessory organs?

_____

_____

3. Name the main organs of digestion.

_____

_____

4. Name the accessory organs of digestion.

_____

C. Circle the correctly spelled word in each of the following statements.

1. Food enters the digestive tract through the (bugle, buccal) cavity.

2. The opening to the mouth is protected by the (labia, labea), or lips.

3. The tongue and its muscles are attached to the floor of the mouth and assist in both chewing and (swallowing, swalowing).

4. The tongue is attached to four bones, the (hyod, hyoid), mandible, and two (tempral, temporal) bones.

5. The taste buds respond to the bitterness, (saltiness, saltyness), sweetness, and (soreness, sourness) in food.

D.   Label the diagram of the mouth and tongue. Color the mucous membrane pink, the gingivae red, the uvula orange, the hard palate yellow, and the soft palate brown.

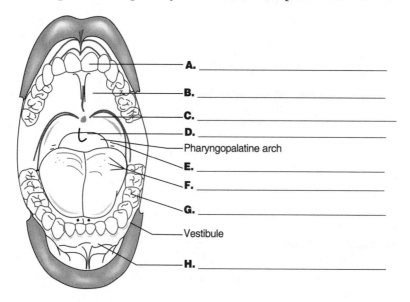

A. _____

B. _____

C. _____

D. _____

Pharyngopalatine arch

E. _____

F. _____

G. _____

Vestibule

H. _____

E.   Using the labels from the previous diagram, match the letter with the following descriptions (letters may be used more than once).

_____   1. This structure is formed from the maxillary and palatine bones.

_____   2. This prevents food from entering the nasal cavity when swallowing.

_____   3. This structure supports and protects the teeth.

_____   4. Nerve endings located here form the taste buds.

F.   Label the salivary glands and state where they are located.

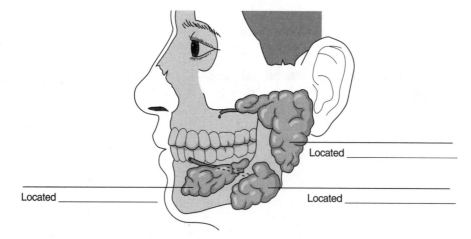

Located _____

Located _____

Located _____

G. Fill in the blanks to complete the following statements.

1. The gland infected in mumps is the _____.

2. The other name for saliva is _____.

3. The salivary glands belong to the _____ system.

4. The _____ salivary gland contains no ptyalin.

H. Label the tooth.

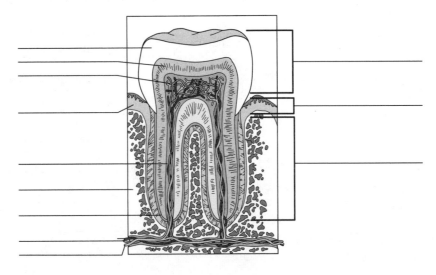

I. Match each term in Column A with a related term in Column B.

Column A	Column B
_____ 1. deciduous	a. mastication
_____ 2. gingivae (gums)	b. sharp edges for biting
_____ 3. chewing	c. support the teeth (gums)
_____ 4. canines	d. eight
_____ 5. number of permanent bicuspids	e. crushing and grinding
_____ 6. incisor teeth	f. milk teeth
_____ 7. number of deciduous canine teeth	g. two
_____ 8. molars	h. tearing and shredding food

J. Fill in the blanks to complete the following statements.

1. The structure that anchors the teeth in place is the _____ membrane.

2. The _____ _____ contains the nerve and blood supply.

3. The hardest substance in the body is _____.

4. The calcified tissue surrounding the pulp cavity is _____.

5. The root of the tooth is embedded in the _____ _____ of the jaw.

K. Mark the following statements either true or false. Correct any false statements.

_____ 1. The esophagus is a muscular tube about 20 inches long, posterior to the trachea.

_____ 2. The esophagus continues from the pharynx through the mediastinum and ends superior to the diaphragm.

_____ 3. The esophagus joins with the cardiac orifice of the stomach.

_____ 4. The muscles in the esophagus are smooth muscles.

L. Label the structures of the stomach. Color the muscle layers three different colors, and the mucosa layer pink. Outline the rugae in black.

M. Compare the following structures.

1. Cardiac sphincter/pyloric sphincter

_____

_____

2. Greater curvature/lesser curvature

_____

_____

3. Pyloric stenosis/pylorospasm

_____

_____

4. Mucosa layer/muscularis layer

_____

_____

N. Complete the following word puzzle, using the clues provided to fill in the missing words regarding the gastric glands.

1. G_____ Stimulates the production of hydrochloric acid and pepsinogen

2. A_____ Mucous type that neutralizes hydrochloric acid

3. S_____ Hydrochloric acid is the body's natural one

G A S T R I C

4. R_____ Found in infants; prepares milk protein

5. I_____ Factor necessary for absorption of vitamin B_{12}

6. C_____ _____ Cells that produce pepsinogen that converts to pepsin

O. Select the letter of the choice that best completes the statement.

1. Pancreatic digestive juices are caused by:
   a. the bloodstream into the duodenum
   b. a duct into the duodenum
   c. the bloodstream into the ileum
   d. a duct into the ileum

2. If the common bile duct is blocked, the skin will become:
   a. cyanotic
   b. jaundiced
   c. ischemic
   d. icteric

3. The liver manufactures all of the following plasma proteins except:
   a. albumin
   b. fibrinogen
   c. prothrombin
   d. hemoglobin

4. The liver prepares urea, the chief waste product of:
   a. protein metabolism
   b. glucose metabolism
   c. fatty acids
   d. glycerol

5. The gallbladder stores bile, which is released when:
   a. foods high in fat enter the stomach
   b. foods with protein content enter the stomach
   c. foods high in fat enter the duodenum
   d. foods low in fat content enter the stomach

6. The large intestine connects with the small intestine at the:
   a. ileocecal valve
   b. pyloric sphincter
   c. cecum
   d. cardiac sphincter

7. The large intestine is:
   a. longer in length and larger in diameter than the small intestine
   b. the same size as the small intestine
   c. shorter in length and larger in diameter than the small intestine
   d. shorter in length but with the same diameter as the small intestine

8. The large intestine is also known as the:
   a. sigmoid
   b. rectum
   c. colon
   d. cecum

9. Below the ileocecal valve is a blind pouch called the:
   a. appendix
   b. cecum
   c. sigmoid
   d. rectum

10. The final structure of the colon is the:
    a. sigmoid colon
    b. descending colon
    c. rectum
    d. anal canal

P. Complete the story about the GI tract using the words from the following list.

amino acid	duodenum	labia	rectum
bile	esophagus	peptones	rugae
buccal	fatty acid	peristalsis	stomach
canines	glucose	protease	tongue
cardiac orifice	hydrochloric acid	ptyalin	uvula
chyme	jejunem	pyloric sphincter	villi
colon			

THE TRIP THROUGH THE GI TRACT

My friends and I decided to try a new ride on the GI tract. I am Taco Corn Chip, and they are Meat and Cheese. We paid admission to Ms. _____ Lips, who looked good enough to kiss, and then entered the GI tract. Standing in the big _____ cavity, all around us were strange white things. They really looked like mad scientists in long white coats, and we were the juicy specimens.

Just then the thick-muscled _____ platform started to move, pushing us up and down toward the white things, which bit and tore at us like angry _____. Next, I was squirted with _____, which came at me through a thin tube and I began to get gooey. I grabbed my friends, who also looked gooey, and we started moving further back in this cavity. "Wait!," someone shouted, "grab your rain gear off the _____ rack, which hangs down from the roof at the rear of the buccal."

Now we are going down the roller coaster called _____ and find ourselves at this strange door marked _____. It slowly opens and we go inside. This _____ room is even stranger; the walls are all draped in _____ folds. Upon our arrival we take a bath using _____ _____; we can now proceed since we are all cleaned up. My friend Meat is hit with _____, which has him singing "I am a peppy little _____," and Cheese is getting softened up. A big voice announces, "You are no longer who you once were. Your name is now _____." Who cares, I think just get me out of here. A big tidal wave called _____ hits just then, pushing us through the exit marked _____ _____.

Now, I am really scared, because this tube goes on forever. We are in the first part of it, the _____. I look around and see a slitlike opening. Look! Cheese is standing right behind me and gets a big squirt of _____ all over him. He is starting to come apart. At this point, we are being hit with all sorts of stuff that breaks us up into strange parts. I transform into _____. Meat is an _____ _____ and Cheese is _____ _____ and glycerol. What will become of us? We get pushed again into the next part of the tunnel, the _____, and our fate is sealed. Awaiting us like a welcome mat are many little fingers called _____. They are now walking right through us, picking us apart. "Goodbye my friends," I shout, as we get sucked up.

There were some pieces of us left over. They were shoved into a bigger tunnel, the _____, where they were dried out and then dumped out through the _____.

RING!! RING!! That is my alarm clock. Oh what a nightmare. I should not have stayed up so late studying for my GI test and stuffing myself with tacos and pizza.

Q. In the following exercise, state what process of digestion takes place in the labeled organs.

1. Mouth: _____

   _____

   _____

2. Salivary glands: _____

   _____

   _____

3. Esophagus: _____

   _____

   _____

4. Stomach: _____

_____

_____

5. Liver: _____

_____

_____

6. Gallbladder: _____

_____

_____

7. Pancreas: _____

_____

_____

8. Small intestine: _____

_____

_____

9. Large intestine: _____

_____

_____

R. Fill in the blanks to complete the following statements on digestion.

1. The passage of food through the digestive tract takes approximately _____ hours; the food is pushed through by _____ and _____ movement.

2. The purpose of the _____ is to cover the _____ to prevent food from entering the trachea.

3. Food takes about _____ to _____ hours to leave the stomach.

4. The large intestines absorb _____, _____, and potassium, which helps in the regulation of _____ balance.

5. The bacterial population of the colon is also referred to as the normal _____.

6. The action of the bacteria on undigested food turns them into _____, _____, and other waste products.

7. Bacteria in the colon help to _____ moderate amounts of vitamins _____ and _____.

8. Gas passed through the rectum is called _____.

9. Cellulose contributes _____ to feces, which _____ the muscular activity of the colon, resulting in _____.

10. When the rectum becomes distended with the accumulation of feces, it triggers the _____ _____. This action results in the relaxation of the _____ _____. For defecation to occur, the _____ _____ must also be relaxed.

S. Match the disorder in Column A with its description in Column B.

Column A	Column B
_____ 1. colitis	a. inflammation of the appendix
_____ 2. enteritis	b. inflammation of the stomach
_____ 3. peritonitis	c. inflammation of the gallbladder
_____ 4. hepatitis	d. inflammation of the colon
_____ 5. stomatitis	e. inflammation of the wall of the colon
_____ 6. gastritis	f. inflammation of the liver
_____ 7. pancreatitis	g. inflammation of the small intestine
_____ 8. cholecystitis	h. inflammation of the peritoneal lining
_____ 9. diverticulitis	i. inflammation of the pancreas
_____ 10. appendicitis	j. inflammation of the soft tissues of the mouth

T. Using words from the following list, complete the statements on digestive disorders.

cirrhosis	heartburn	histamine	pyloric stenosis
constipation	hepatitis A	*H. pylori*	stomach cancer
Crohn's disease	hepatitis B	gallstones	stress
diarrhea	hiatal hernia	gastroesophageal reflux	ulcer
diverticula			

1. Many symptoms of digestive problems are caused by _____.

2. When the sphincter muscle is weak and the stomach contents flow up into the esophagus, the condition is _____.

3. _____ _____ occurs in many people over age 50, the stomach protrudes above the diaphragm.

4. A backflow of the acidic gastric juices causes indigestion or _____.

5. A narrowing of the sphincter at the lower end of the stomach causing projectile vomiting is _____ _____.

6. A lesion that occurs in the lining of the stomach or small intestine is an _____.

7. Research shows that most ulcers are caused by the bacteria _____.

8. Drugs that reduce the amount of acid produced by the stomach are called _____ blockers.

9. Chronic dehydration, ulceration of the bowel, and personal embarrassment are symptoms of _____ _____.

10. _____ is a viral infection of the liver, spread through contaminated food and water; enteric precautions must be followed.

11. _____ is a viral infection of the liver, spread through contaminated blood; standard precautions must be taken at all times of exposure.

12. Liver disease, characterized by replacement of the normal tissue with fibrotic connective tissue, usually caused by excessive consumption of alcohol, is known as _____.

13. The majority of people over the age of 60 have little sacs, called _____, that develop in the wall of the colon.

14. Loose, watery bowel movements that can lead to dehydration are called _____.

15. A condition of hardened stool that can be caused by anxiety, fear, or fright, is known as _____.

16. The treatment of _____ _____ may also lead to pernicious anemia.

U. Find the following words relating to the digestive system in the puzzle.

```
s d p e x m j s n b i l e d m u c e c l d y a r
p i e a s i u e i i a k d r e c l u e i o b e x
a a s f x o d n j g s f e c e s q m g u s d s d
o m n l e g p n e u m p c x h z a e r o d i i e
w z y c a c r h e d n o e o f n s e r a t a a s
l e r l r t a e a p o u i p e t t p l i r v i o
a v e e a e s t t g p u m d i c t b t r i t m c
n l c e s s a i i c u a d o n i l a h g i e a c
a a t r l a e s r o n s n i o l p e n l n n h h
c v u j i s p x r e n i h n a e a i o t i s v y
y l m x v o v i k f p p h g h d g c u n w w u m
r a a m e u i j l g s b c p h m e m e z o e a e
a c n u r r u m s c u z c o s e a c d t h e l v
t e u e q z o i a c c m i i n c a s i e q t u t
n c s l q l t i c o e n j p r s i r t d n g v l
e o t i a i d a s s t a r s q r t r t i u t u a
n e a r r r l d e r u o y p t s h i o b c o i s
i l s t a c i n i n t r h c a e r o p l u a u n
l i s c a p t n d e a c h p z p a o s a y r t s
a a b v s e s i a v a f D R E G i p s i t p n e
g o i u r i c s i m v i l l i d q l s i s i s i
n t c y c e e l o c o l o n q k f y l i c r o n
y i p w y p a t t e t s a t s u l o b a n n a n
b a r u h s s i n t r i n s i c f a c t o r i z
```

absorption	hepatitis
alimentary	illeocecal valve
canal	ileum
amylase	incisors
anus	intrinsic
appendix	factor
biscuspids	jaundice
bile	jejunum
bolus	lipase
buccal cavity	liver
canine	masticate
cardiac	mesentery
sphincter	molars
cecum	omentum
chyme	pancreas
cirrhosis	papilla
colitis	pepsin
colon	peristalsis
constipation	protease
deciduous	pyloric
defecation	sphincter
dentin	rectum
diarrhea	salivary
digestion	salt
duodenum	sigmoid
enamel	sour
esophagus	steapsin
feces	stomach
gallbladder	sweet
gastritis	taste
GERD	ulcer
gingivae	uvula
heartburn	villi

APPLYING THEORY TO PRACTICE

1. Career opportunities exist in the field of dentistry. Prepare a career exploration seminar for junior high school students describing the jobs of dentists, dental hygienists, dental assistants, and dental laboratory technicians.

_____

_____

_____

_____

_____

_____

_____

_____

_____

2. A friend is thinking of becoming a health care worker, but she is concerned about hepatitis. She wants to know her chances of contracting the disease. Explain hepatitis, the various types, and to which types health care workers may be exposed. What is the current recommendation for workers in the health care field?

_____

_____

_____

_____

_____

3. Because so many people have episodes of heartburn, there are many remedies for this problem. Describe the latest over-the-counter nonprescription treatment for this problem. How does it differ from other antacid preparations?

_____

_____

_____

_____

4. The treatment for cancer of the colon frequently involves colostomy surgery. What are some of the difficulties patients have in accepting this procedure? How can you relieve some of this anxiety?

_____

_____

_____

_____

5. Keisha goes to the dentist because her gums bleed when she brushes her teeth. What is causing her gums to bleed? What can this problem lead to and how can it be prevented? What is the function of the teeth and periodontal membrane?

_____

_____

_____

_____

6. Linda has been losing weight and decides to visit her physician. After doing abdominal sonograms, the doctor suspects cancer of the stomach. Linda is distressed and questions the doctor regarding the lack of her symptoms. What responses does the doctor give Linda? How is cancer of the stomach treated and what is the prognosis?

_____

_____

_____

_____

7. Eileen is being treated for peptic ulcer. Her doctor suggests an endoscopy as a follow-up examination to be certain the ulcer has healed. Eileen has heard about a new technique for taking pictures of the digestive system and asks Lauren, the medical assistant, about this procedure. What information should Lauren give Eileen regarding how the swallowable camera works?

Where do peptic ulcers occur? What is the treatment for peptic ulcers?

_____

_____

_____

_____

8. Hector, age 75, has been complaining to Daniel, the health care worker at the senior center, that he has a problem with constipation. Hector tells Daniel that in the past, fruit was very effective in producing regular bowel movements. What information does Daniel need to give Hector regarding how aging affects the process of defecation?

_____

_____

_____

_____

SURF THE NET

Briefly summarize your findings from the Web sites given, or choose alternate sites for the following topics.

1. For a quiz on the anatomy of the digestive system, go to
   http://www.gen.umn.edu/faculty_staff/jensen/1135/webanatomy/wa_digestive/

2. For facts on periodontal disease, go to
   http://www.fda.gov/fdac/features/2002/302_gums.html

3. How much do you know about stomach ulcers? Find out at,
   http://www.principalhealthnews.com/topic/ulcerquiz;$essionid$N

4. For information on hepatitis C, go to http://www.hep-help.com/treat/index.html

Nutrition

OVERVIEW

Nutrients

Nutrients are materials needed by the individual cells for optimal cell functioning. Nutrients include water, carbohydrates, lipids, proteins, vitamins, and minerals.

Water makes up about 55% to 60% of the body. It is an essential component of body tissue. Its functions include:

Acting as a solvent for all biochemical reactions.

Serving as a transport medium for substances.

Lubricating joint movement and the digestive tract.

Controlling body temperature.

Serving as a cushion for the lungs and the brain.

Carbohydrates include the simple and complex sugars. They are the main source of energy for the body.

A **calorie** is a unit that measures the amount of energy contained within the chemical bonds. A small calorie is the amount of heat needed to raise the temperature of 1 gram of water by 1°C.

Lipids or **fats** are a group of compounds of fatty acids combined with an alcohol. They are a storehouse of energy, cushion internal organs, insulate against cold, and contain the fat-soluble vitamins A, D, E, and K.

Cholesterol is a fat found in animal products, including milk, meat, and cheese. It is a white, wax-like substance used to build cells and make hormones. If cholesterol builds up in the body, it causes atherosclerosis. The high-density lipoprotein, HDL, helps to remove excess cholesterol.

Proteins are more complex than carbohydrates and fats and contain an amino group. They are synthesized in the cell cytoplasm from constituent molecules called amino acids. Proteins are important in the growth and repair of body tissue and make up the enzymes that regulate the rate of chemical reactions. They cannot be stored and are excreted as urea.

Minerals, trace elements, and **vitamins** are necessary for normal growth and maintenance of the body.

Mineral: chemical element that is obtained from inorganic compounds in food such as sodium, potassium, and so forth

Trace elements: present in the body in small amounts (e.g., zinc; see Table 19-2 in your textbook).

Vitamin: biologically active organic compound (see Table 19-3 in your textbook).

Fiber is found only in plant foods, such as whole-grain breads and fruit. It is important to include fiber in the diet for normal bowel functioning.

Effects of Aging

Chronic disease, social, economic, physical, and emotional factors affect the diet of the elderly.

The **Recommended Dietary Allowances (RDA)** contain the daily recommendations for the protein, fat-soluble, and water-soluble vitamins and minerals.

Basal metabolic rate is the measure of the total energy utilized by the body to maintain body processes that are necessary for life.

Dietary guidelines for Americans are shown in the food guide pyramid, which recommends the food necessary to provide essential nutrients.

Nutritional labeling must include information on total calories from a variety of foods.

Food poisoning occurs when microscopic organisms grow in food undetected and then cause illness after they are eaten.

Eating Disorders

Obesity.   If a person's weight is 15% more than the optimum body weight for gender, height, and bone structure, then he or she is considered obese.

Anorexia Nervosa.   Anorexia nervosa is a refusal to eat because of a distorted body image and fear of weight gain.

Bulimia.   Bulimia is an episodic binge eating followed by behavior such as self-induced vomiting, which the bulimic believes will maintain body weight.

ACTIVITIES

A.   Fill in the blanks to complete the following statements.

1. For our cells to function properly, they need _____.

2. These materials include _____, _____, _____, _____, _____, and _____.

3. Water is lost in the body through _____, _____, and _____.

B.   Answer the following questions relating to nutrients.

1. Name five important functions of water.

_____

_____

_____

_____

_____

2. Describe the functions of carbohydrates, fats, and proteins.

_____

_____

_____

C. Water makes up between 55% and 65% of our total body weight. Calculate the water weight of the following:

1. A person weighing 200 pounds, with 62% water weight

_____

2. A person weighing 140 pounds, with 57% water weight

_____

3. A person weighing 90 pounds, with 60% water weight

_____

D. Select the letter of the choice that best completes the statement.

1. The recommended dietary intake of carbohydrates is:
   a. 40% to 50% of the daily intake of calories
   b. 50% to 60% of the daily intake of calories
   c. 60% to 70% of the daily intake of calories
   d. 70% to 80% of the daily intake of calories

2. Five grams of fat equal:
   a. 45 calories
   b. 36 calories
   c. 25 calories
   d. 24 calories

3. A female is 24 years old, weighs 128 pounds, and is 65 inches tall; she is also 4 months pregnant. Her daily requirement for calories will be:
   a. 2,000 calories
   b. 2,200 calories
   c. 2,500 calories
   d. 2,800 calories

4. A 50-year-old male weighs 174 pounds and is 70 inches tall. His daily requirement for calories will be:
   a. 1,500 calories
   b. 2,500 calories
   c. 1,800 calories
   d. 2,000 calories

5. Starch and cellulose provide all of the following except:
   a. roughage
   b. minerals
   c. empty calories
   d. vitamins

6. Glycolipid is an example of a:
   a. simple lipid
   b. compound lipid
   c. cholesterol
   d. carbohydrates

7. Excess protein is:
   a. eliminated by the body
   b. stored in the body as an amino acid
   c. stored in the body as fat
   d. stored in the body as a complete protein

8. The good lipoprotein that removes excess cholesterol is:
   a. VLDL
   b. LDL
   c. HDL
   d. LTH

9. An example of a polyunsaturated fat is:
   a. butter
   b. olive oil
   c. sunflower oil
   d. peanut oil

10. All of the following foods help lower cholesterol except:
   a. olive oil
   b. peanut oil
   c. safflower oil
   d. cheese

E. Answer the following questions regarding foods, minerals, and vitamins.

1. If your diet included all of the following foods, listed in E-2, would it meet your nutritional needs? Are all the essential amino acids present?

   _____

   _____

   _____

2. When your menu includes the following foods, which minerals and vitamins are being provided? Fill in the table.

Food	Mineral	Vitamin
a. milk	_____	_____
b. cheese	_____	_____
c. eggs	_____	_____
d. green leafy vegetables	_____	_____
e. table salt	_____	_____
f. liver	_____	_____
g. meat	_____	_____
h. poultry	_____	_____
i. fish	_____	_____
j. shellfish	_____	_____
k. shrimp	_____	_____
l. yellow vegetables	_____	_____
m. legumes	_____	_____
n. fruit	_____	_____
o. molasses	_____	_____
p. drinking water	_____	_____
q. cherries	_____	_____
r. nuts	_____	_____

F. Match the mineral in Column A with the result of a deficiency in that mineral in Column B. Use each item in Column B only once.

Column A	Column B
_____ 1. calcium	a. muscular weakness
_____ 2. chlorine	b. deficiency in amino acid
_____ 3. chromium	c. muscular cramps
_____ 4. copper	d. weakness
_____ 5. fluorine	e. demineralization of the bone
_____ 6. iodine	f. lack of sexual maturity
_____ 7. iron	g. behavioral disturbance
_____ 8. magnesium	h. impaired ability to metabolize glucose
_____ 9. phosphorous	i. anemia
_____ 10. potassium	j. deficiency is rare
_____ 11. selenium	k. goiter
_____ 12. sodium	l. convulsions
_____ 13. sulfur	m. iron-deficiency anemia
_____ 14. zinc	n. tooth decay

G. List vitamins necessary for each of the following:

1. Normal bone and teeth   _____

2. Normal blood clotting   _____

3. Nucleic acid synthesis   _____

4. Cellular respiration   _____

5. Night vision   _____

6. Nervous system   _____

7. Normal growth   _____

8. Red blood cell synthesis   _____

H. Complete the table on vitamins.

VITAMIN	FOOD SOURCES	FUNCTION	DEFICIENCY DISEASES
_____ _____	Butter, fortified margarine, green and yellow vegetables, milk, eggs, liver	_____ _____ _____ _____	Night blindness Dry skin Slow growth Poor gums and teeth
B$_1$ (thiamine) (Water soluble)	Chicken, fish, meat, eggs, enriched bread, whole-grain cereals	_____ _____ _____ _____	_____ _____ _____
_____ _____	_____ _____ _____	Needed in cellular respiration	_____ _____
B$_3$ (niacin) (Water soluble)	Eggs, fish, liver, meat, milk, potatoes, enriched bread	_____ _____ _____ _____	Indigestion Diarrhea Headaches Mental disturbances Skin disorders
_____ _____ _____	Milk, liver, brain, beef, egg yolk, clams, oysters, sardines, salmon	_____ _____ _____	_____ _____
_____ _____	Liver, yeast, green vegetables, peanuts, mushrooms, beef, veal, egg yolk	_____ _____	_____ _____
_____ _____	Citrus fruits, cabbage, green vegetables, tomatoes, potatoes	_____ _____ _____	_____ _____ _____ _____ _____ _____

VITAMIN	FOOD SOURCES	FUNCTION	DEFICIENCY DISEASES
_____ _____	_____	Needed for normal bone and teeth development Controls calcium and phosphorus metabolism	Poor bone and teeth structure Soft bones Rickets
_____ _____	Margarine, nuts, leafy vegetables, vegetable oils, whole wheat	_____ _____ _____	_____ _____
_____ _____	Synthesized by colon bacteria Green leafy vegetables, cereal	_____ _____	_____ _____

I. Mark the following statements as either true or false. Correct any false statements.

_____ 1. According to the food pyramid, the recommended bread intake per day is 6 to 11 servings.

_____ 2. According to the food pyramid, the number of daily fruit servings should be 3 to 5 servings.

_____ 3. When we experience stress, we need a lesser amount of certain nutrients to maintain homeostasis.

_____ 4. Nutrition labels include information and total calories listed in a specific order.

_____ 5. The amount of each nutrient as a percentage of the recommended daily values is based on a 2,500-calorie diet.

_____ 6. The definition of obese is 10% over the optimum body weight for gender, height, and bone structure of a particular person.

_____ 7. In anorexia nervosa, there is a loss of appetite.

_____ 8. Bulimia is characterized by episodic binge eating followed by induced vomiting.

_____ 9. Tooth-friendly cheeses are cheddar, Swiss, Edam, and Gouda.

_____10. Barley may be an effective food to lower cholesterol.

APPLYING THEORY TO PRACTICE

1. A person has an intake of 3,100 calories per day. If 25% is fat and 15% is protein, what percentage is carbohydrates? How many grams of fat, protein, and carbohydrate are in this diet?

_____

_____

2. Your friend is a vegetarian and has iron-deficiency anemia. Recommend a diet that will meet her needs.

_____

_____

_____

3. Read the labels on the following and indicate the daily requirements met in each of these foods, in an average serving.

   a. Box of cereal _____

   _____

   b. Candy bar _____

   _____

   c. Loaf of bread _____

   _____

   d. Frozen vegetables _____

   _____

   e. Quart of ice cream _____

   _____

4. Much has been written about the healing power of foods. What foods are thought to be good in lowering cholesterol, fighting tooth decay, helping with arthritis, and preventing colds?

   _____

   _____

   _____

5. Dominick is 17 years old and has a family history of heart disease; he asks the school nutritionist, Kayla, what dietary guidelines can he follow to reduce his risk of heart disease. Explain the guidelines Kayla can give Dominick to reduce the risk.

   _____

   _____

   _____

6. Margaret had lunch with her 3-year-old son at a fast-food restaurant. After a few hours they both experienced flulike symptoms. Margaret thought they might have had a touch of food poisoning. What can Carolyn, the medical assistant, tell Margaret about safety factors regarding food?

   _____

   _____

   _____

7. Calculate the BMR for Kreg, an active 40-year-old male who is 5′10″ and weighs 170 pounds. Calculate Kreg's BMI; is it within normal limits?

_____

_____

_____

SURF THE NET

Briefly summarize your findings from the suggested Web sites, or choose alternate sites for the following topics.

1. To find out how sports drinks measure up to the fitness test, go to
   http://www.monash.edu.au/pubs/montage/Montage_96-05/Sportdrink.html

2. Do you know your vitamin ABCs? Go to http://www.principalhealthnews.com/topic/vitquiz

3. For facts on fitness and nutrition, go to http://www.principalhealthnews.com/topic/fitness

4. How much do you know about cold food storage? Go to
   http://www.vdacs.state.va.us/foodsafety/refrigquiz.html

Urinary/Excretory System

OVERVIEW

The **urinary/excretory system** includes those organs that eliminate waste products. **Elimination of waste products** is through the following:

Kidneys excrete nitrogenous waste, salts, and water through urination, and maintain the acid-base balance.

Skin excretes water and salt through perspiration.

Intestines excrete indigestible food, water, and bacteria through defecation.

Lungs excrete carbon dioxide and water vapor through exhalation.

Urinary System

The organs of the urinary system include two kidneys, two ureters, a bladder, and a urethra.

Kidneys. The kidneys are two bean-shaped organs located in the retroperitoneal area.

Adipose capsule is a mass of fat tissues that encloses the kidney and blood vessels.

Renal fascia is fibrous tissue that covers the adipose capsule.

Hilum is an indentation along the medial border; serves as a passageway for lymph vessels, nerves, artery, and vein.

Renal pelvis is a funnel-shaped structure at the upper end of each ureter.

The kidney is divided into two layers. The outer granular layer is called the cortex and the inner striated layer is called the medulla.

The **cortex** consists of millions of functional units called *nephrons.*

The **medulla** consists of renal pyramids, whose apexes empty into cuplike structures (calyces) which in turn empty into the renal pelvis.

Nephron. The nephron is the structural and functional unit of the kidney. It begins with the afferent arteriole, which carries blood from the renal artery to *Bowman's capsule,* a double-walled, hollow structure. Within the capsule, the arteriole divides, forming a ball of capillaries called the *glomerulus,* and then leaves the area as the *efferent arteriole* and forms the *capillary network* around the tubules.

Proximal convoluted tubule is a twisted tubular branch extending from the Bowman's capsule.

Loop of Henle is a proximal convoluted tubule that descends and forms a loop (the loop descends into the medulla part of the kidney).

Distal convoluted tubule is where the ascending loop of Henle returns to the cortex of the kidney.

Collecting tubule is a straight collection tubule that empties into the renal pelvis and then into the ureter.

In **urine formation in the nephron,** the nephron uses three processes: filtration by the glomerulus, reabsorption within the renal tubules, and secretion by the tubular cells.

In *filtration,* blood enters the afferent arteriole and plasmalike fluid filters from the blood into the glomerulus, then through Bowman's capsule. The fluid, called filtrate, does not contain red blood cells or plasma proteins.

In *reabsorption,* substances are reabsorbed as they pass through the tubules. Proximal tubules reabsorb 80% of the water filtered out of the blood in the glomerulus, called obligatory reabsorption. Other substances are also reabsorbed.

In the loop of Henle and distal tubule, substances continue to be absorbed. In the distal tubules another 10% to 15% of water is reabsorbed, which is called optimal reabsorption. This process is controlled by ADH and aldosterone.

In *secretion,* the opposite of reabsorption, substances secreted are ammonia, hydrogen, and potassium ions. If a person is taking medication, the drugs may also be secreted.

The following is the **path of urine formation:** Blood enters the afferent arteriole, passing through the glomerulus to Bowman's capsule, as filtrate. It continues through the proximal convoluted tubule to the loop of Henle, on to the distal convoluted tubule, the collecting tubules, the renal pelvis, the ureter, the bladder, the urethra, and finally the urinary meatus.

Urinary output is on average, approximately 1,500 to 2,400 ml/day. One milliliter of urine is formed per minute.

Ureters. The ureters are two narrow tubes running from the renal pelvis to the bladder.

Urinary Bladder. The urinary bladder acts like a reservoir, storing urine until approximately 500 ml is accumulated; the act of urination then occurs.

Urethra. The urethra is a narrow canal running from the bladder to the outside urinary meatus.

Control of Urinary Secretion

Chemical Control. Chemical control includes hormones that promote reabsorption in the distal convoluted tubules, namely, aldosterone and ADH.

Aldosterone promotes the excretion of potassium and reabsorption of sodium, which causes reabsorption of water. As blood passes through Bowman's capsule, receptors can detect a drop in blood pressure. Renin is then released by the capsule into the bloodstream, which triggers the release of aldosterone (from the adrenal cortex).

ADH is released when the osmoreceptors in the hypothalamus detect an increase in the osmotic blood pressure due to salt retention. This causes an increase in the reabsorption of water in the tubules

Nervous Control. Nervous control is accomplished directly through the action of nerve impulses on the blood vessels leading to the kidney and on those within the kidney leading to the urethra.

Effects of Aging

There is a decrease in nephrons and glomerular filtration rate, which results a decrease in renal blood flow. This compromises the ability of the kidney to eliminate waste. Loss of muscle tone leads to urinary incontinence and nocturia.

Disorders of the Urinary System

Acute kidney failure is caused by nephritis, shock, injury, bleeding, sudden heart failure, or poisoning; symptoms include oliguria and anuria.

Uremia is a toxic condition in which the blood retains urinary waste products because the kidneys fail to excrete them.

Chronic renal failure is a gradual loss of function of the nephrons.

Glomerulonephritis is inflammation of the glomerulus of the nephron.

Acute glomerulonephritis usually occurs in children, 1 to 3 weeks after a bacterial infection.

Chronic glomerulonephritis may permanently affect the filtration membrane.

Hydronephrosis results in renal pelvis and calyces becoming distended due to an accumulation of fluid.

Pyelitis is an inflammation of the pelvis of the kidney.

Pyelonephritis is an inflammation of the kidney tissue along with its renal pelvis.

Kidney stones are also called renal calculi; stones form in the kidney.

Lithotripsy is the use of ultrasound techniques to pulverize the stone which then may be passed in the urine.

Cystitis is inflammation of the mucous membrane lining of the urinary bladder, leading to dysuria and polyuria.

Neurogenic bladder is caused by a damaged nerve that controls the urinary bladder.

Urethritis is inflammation of the urethra.

Dialysis.   Dialysis is the passage of dissolved molecules through a semipermeable membrane. This treatment serves as a substitute kidney.

Hemodialysis: Blood is removed from an artery, passes through a dialyzer, and is returned to a vein.

Peritoneal dialysis: The peritoneal membrane acts as the semipermeable membrane.

Kidney Transplants.   Kidney transplants require a donor organ from an individual who has a similar immune system to prevent rejection.

ACTIVITIES

A. Answer the following questions on the urinary system.

1. Name the excretory organs and the waste products they excrete.

_____

_____

_____

_____

_____

_____

2. Describe the function of the urinary system.

_____

_____

_____

_____

_____

B. Label the structures of the urinary system.

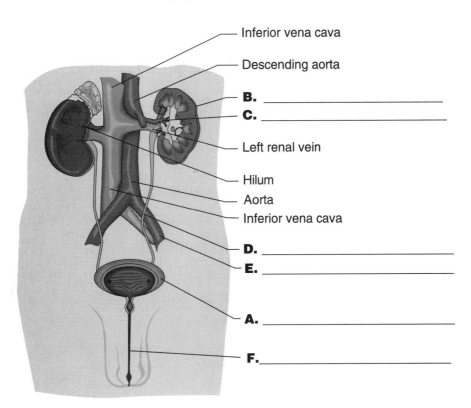

Inferior vena cava

Descending aorta

B. _____

C. _____

Left renal vein

Hilum

Aorta

Inferior vena cava

D. _____

E. _____

A. _____

F. _____

C. Using the previous figure, match the letter of the function to each structure.

_____ 1. Takes urine to the outside of the body

_____ 2. Organ that removes nitrogenous waste

_____ 3. Stores urine

_____ 4. Brings blood to the kidney

_____ 5. Brings blood to the urinary bladder

_____ 6. Transports urine from kidney to bladder

D. Select the letter of the choice that best completes the statement.

1. Kidneys are said to be retroperitoneal, which means they are:
   a. located inside the peritoneal cavity
   b. located behind the peritoneal cavity
   c. lie on either side of the vertebrae
   d. rest high against the dorsal wall of the abdominal cavity

2. Each kidney is covered with a tough fibrous tissue called the:
   a. adipose capsule
   b. omentum
   c. renal fasciae
   d. mesentery

3. The upper end of each ureter flares into a(n):
   a. funnel-shaped structure, the pelvis
   b. outer granular layer, the cortex
   c. long tube called the urethra
   d. concave medial border, the hilum

4. The kidney is divided internally into the medulla and cortex. The medulla consists of individually striated cones called the:
   a. renal pyramids
   b. pelvis
   c. renal papillae
   d. calyces

5. Cuplike structures that empty into the renal pelvis are known as:
   a. renal pyramids
   b. renal papillae
   c. renal calyces
   d. renal fascia

6. The outer part of the kidney, the cortex, consists of:
   a. pyramids
   b. papillae
   c. calyces
   d. nephrons

7. The blood pressure in most of the capillaries in the body is 25 ml of mercury; in the glomerulus it is:
   a. 30 to 60 ml
   b. 60 to 90 ml
   c. 90 to 120 ml
   d. 120 to 150 ml

8. Obligatory reabsorption of water by osmosis is when:
   a. 60% is absorbed in the proximal convoluted tubule
   b. 70% is absorbed in the proximal convoluted tubule
   c. 80% is absorbed in the proximal convoluted tubule
   d. 90% is absorbed in the proximal convoluted tubule

9. Optimal reabsorption takes place in the:
   a. Bowman's capsule
   b. glomerulus
   c. proximal convoluted tubule
   d. distal convoluted tubule

10. The Bowman's capsule filters 125 ml of fluid per minute; 99% of the fluid is reabsorbed. How much filtrate is produced per minute?
    a. 1 ml
    b. 2 ml
    c. 12.5 ml
    d. 7.5 ml

E. Label the structure of the nephron. Color the glomerulus red; Bowman's capsule and proximal convoluted tubule yellow; the loop of Henle distal convoluted tubule, and collecting tubules orange.

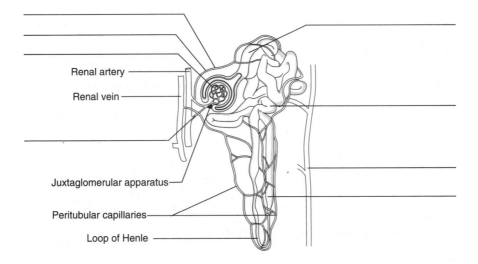

Renal artery

Renal vein

Juxtaglomerular apparatus

Peritubular capillaries

Loop of Henle

F.   Describe the structures and functions of the following:

1. Afferent arteriole

   _____

   _____

2. Glomerulus

   _____

   _____

3. Efferent arteriole

   _____

   _____

4. Bowman's capsule

   _____

   _____

5. Proximal convoluted tubule

   _____

   _____

6. Loop of Henle

   _____

   _____

7. Distal convoluted tubule

   _____

   _____

8. Collecting tubule

   _____

   _____

G.   List substances added or removed during the following actions.

1. Tubular filtration   _____

   _____

2. Tubular reabsorption _____

   _____

3. Tubular secretion _____

_____

H. Answer the following questions.

1. Name the factors that affect urinary output.

_____

_____

_____

2. Urine is formed by what three processes?

_____

_____

I. Using the words from the following list, complete the statements regarding the formation of urine. Words may be used more than once.

ADH	filtrate	peritubular capillaries
afferent arteriole	glomerulus	proximal convoluted
blood	glycosuria	plasma protein
Bowman's capsule	increase	red blood cell
collecting tubule	loop of Henle	renal artery
decrease	obligatory	renal vein
distal convoluted tubule	optional	therapeutic
exceeds	osmosis	threshold
125 ml	100 ml	7,500 ml
80	10–15	60%

1. Blood from the _____ _____ goes to the _____ _____ which then becomes a ball of capillaries, the _____.

2. The blood vessels become narrower leaving the renal artery, which results in an _____ in blood pressure in the capillaries.

3. This action forces blood from the _____ into _____ _____. The fluid is now called a _____.

4. The filtrate contains all the elements of the blood except _____ _____ and _____ _____ _____.

5. Bowman's capsule filters about _____ _____ of fluid from the blood in 1 minute, about _____ _____ of filtrate per hour.

6. Reabsorption begins in the _____ _____ tubule (a continuation of the Bowman's capsule) and continues through the _____ _____ _____, _____ _____ tubule, and the collecting tubule.

7. The proximal tubules reabsorb _____ % of water filtered out of the _____ .

8. This is considered _____ water absorption by _____, the fluid the body needs to survive.

9. The selective cells lining the tubules and the loop of Henle reabsorb other material until a certain level is reached. The term used to describe this level is _____. Passing the level is referred to as spilling over the level.

10. For example glucose is absorbed until the _____ is reached, above which it will no longer be absorbed and _____ occurs. This may also explain why some medications must be taken several times daily to maintain a _____ dosage of the drug in the blood.

11. The _____ _____ tubule reabsorbs _____ – _____ percent of water, depending on the needs of the body. This is called _____ reabsorption, which is controlled by _____ .

12. Secretion, the opposite of reabsorption, transports material from the blood in the _____ _____ into the distal convoluted tubule, which then is added to the filtrate, then passed on to the collecting tubules.

J. Circle the correctly spelled word in each of the following statements.

1. The smooth muscles of the (ureter, uretre) contract, (initialing, initiating) peristalsis, and urine is pushed from the pelvis of the kidney to the bladder.

2. The urinary bladder is a hollow muscular organ that acts like a (resevoir, reservoir) and stores urine.

3. When 500 ml of urine (accumulate, acumulate), the bladder must be emptied.

4. (Voiding, Voieding) is the act of urination.

5. The (reabsorbtion, reabsorption) of water in the distal convoluted tubule is (influenced, influinced) by ADH.

6. ADH increases the size of the cell membrane pores in the distal convoluted tubules which increases the (permebility, permeability) to water.

7. The (osmoticreceptors, osmoreceptors) in the hypothalamus are sensitive to the osmotic blood pressure of the blood plasma. An increase in the osmotic blood pressure due to salt retention causes an increase in ADH which inhibits normal water retention.

8. Aldosterone promotes the (excretion, escretion) of potassium and hydrogen ions and the reabsorption of sodium, chloride, and water ions.

9. The hormone renin is (released, relesed) by the kidneys and into the bloodstream when the cells in Bowman's capsule detect a drop in blood pressure. Renin stimulates the release of aldosterone from the adrenal gland.

10. Any (disfunction, dysfunction) of the adrenal cortex produces pronounced changes in the salt and water content of body fluids.

K. Mark the following statements as either true or false. Correct any false statements.

_____ 1. A major symptom of acute kidney failure is oliguria, which is the absence of urine formation.

_____ 2. Uremia is a toxic condition that occurs when the blood retains urinary waste products.

_____ 3. In chronic renal failure, there is a gradual loss of function of the nephron.

_____ 4. Glomerulonephritis may be acute or chronic; in both conditions, protein is found in the urine.

_____ 5. Hydronephrosis occurs when the renal pelvis and calyces become distended due to an accumulation of fluid; this condition may occur 1 to 3 weeks after a bacterial infection.

_____ 6. An inflammation of the kidney tissue in the renal pelvis is pyelonephritis.

_____ 7. Renal calculi are accumulations of crystals of calcium phosphate, which clump together and may fill the renal papillae.

_____ 8. Diagnostic tests for kidney disease include KUB and IVP.

_____ 9. Treatment for kidney stones includes decreased fluid intake, medication to dissolve stones, and lithotripsy if necessary.

_____ 10. The most common cause of cystitis is *E. coli.* Symptoms include dysuria and polyuria.

_____ 11. Ureteritis is an inflammation of the urethra.

_____ 12. Incontinence is also known as involuntary urination, which occurs in stroke patients and babies.

L. Match the disorder in Column A with the treatment in Column B.

Column A	Column B
_____ 1. acute kidney failure	a. antibiotics
_____ 2. hydronephrosis	b. increasing fluids
_____ 3. pyelonephritis	c. proper hygienic techniques
_____ 4. kidney stones	d. removal of obstruction
_____ 5. cystitis	e. dialysis

M. Fill in the blanks to complete the following statements regarding dialysis.

1. Dialysis involves the passage of blood through a _____, which has a _____ membrane to rid the body of harmful wastes.

2. In hemodialysis, substances in the blood pass through the membranes into the lesser concentrated _____ in response to the laws of _____.

3. The patient is connected to the dialysis unit by means of a _____ or _____, which are surgical constructions to provide a site for inserting the needle.

4. Dialysis is usually done _____ to _____ times per week and lasts from _____ to _____ hours.

5. The patient on dialysis must take medications and follow a _____ diet.

6. In peritoneal dialysis, the person's own _____ lining is used to filter the blood.

7. In peritoneal dialysis, a _____ solution fills the abdominal cavity. Fluid and waste material pass into the _____ from tiny blood vessels in the peritoneal membrane.

8. The most common type of peritoneal dialysis is continuous ambulatory peritoneal dialysis. The dialysate stays in the abdomen for about _____ to _____ hours and is then drained from the abdomen.

9. In kidney transplant, a donor organ must be obtained from a person who has a _____ _____ system.

10. The major complication in kidney transplant is _____.

N. Use the stem to make a new word that fits the definition.

1. _____uria   painful urination
2. _____uria   scanty urine
3. _____uria   little or no urine
4. _____uria   too much urine
5. _____uria   blood in the urine
6. _____uria   protein in the urine
7. _____uria   pus in the urine
8. _____uria   sugar in the urine

APPLYING THEORY TO PRACTICE

1. If a patient had a urinalysis done and plasma proteins and red blood cells were shown in the urine, it would indicate a problem with what part of the nephron?

_____

_____

2. What is the advantage of doing a urinalysis over other diagnostic tests?

_____

_____

3. In glomerular filtration, how much filtrate passes through in 6, 10, and 15 hours?

_____

_____

4. A friend has kidney disease and may need dialysis. He wants to know exactly what the kidney does regarding blood purification. Explain by using the path in the formation of urine as your guide.

_____

_____

_____

_____

5. Margaret is pregnant and she seems to be having a kidney problem. What kidney disorder is common in pregnant women? What is the reason for a common urinary infection in females? Explain the condition and how to prevent it.

_____

_____

SURF THE NET

Briefly summarize your findings from the suggested Web sites, or choose alternate sites for the following topics.

1. To discover how your kidney works, go to
    http://www.howstuffworks.lycoszone.com/kidney/4.htm

2. For information about kidney and urinary problems, go to
    http://www.principalhealthnews.com/topic/kidney

3. For updates on diabetes and kidney disease, go to
    http://www.jdf.org/living_w_diabetes/pages/kidney.php

Reproductive System

OVERVIEW

Reproduction is the act of reproducing a new member of the species; in humans this is done by sexual intercourse.

Function of the Reproductive System. Functions of the reproductive system include (1) the necessary organs capable of reproduction; and (2) the production of hormones necessary for the development of the reproductive organs and the secondary sex characteristics. The hormones are estrogen and progesterone in the female and testosterone in the male.

Reproduction Process. In the reproduction process, the *germ cells*, or *gametes*, are ova in the female and sperm in the male. Normal cell division is mitosis, a duplication of the 46 chromosomes. In human reproduction, meiosis occurs. *Meiosis* reduces the number of chromosomes in the germ cells to 23; when the ova and sperm unite, the fertilized egg contains 46 chromosomes, the same number as the other cells of the body.

Fertilization. In fertilization, the sperm is deposited in the vagina and travels up through the uterus to the fallopian tube. One milliliter of semen contains 100 million sperm. For fertilization to occur, the epithelial cells around the ova must be broken down. Hundreds of sperm swarming produce the enzyme necessary to penetrate the cells. One sperm then unites with the egg. Fertilization, the union of the sperm nucleus with the ovum nucleus to form a fertilized egg or *zygote*, occurs in the outer one-third of the fallopian tube. The ovum has two X sex chromosomes; the sperm has an X and a Y sex chromosome. In reproduction, a female comes from the union of two X chromosomes, the male from an X and Y chromosome. The male parent determines the sex of the child.

Fetal Development. The zygote travels through the fallopian tube and implants itself into the endometrial lining of the uterus and fetal development continues. See Table 21-1 for phases of fetal development and embryonic germ layers.

The female and male sex organs develop from the same embryonic tissue. For the first 2 months there is no gender difference; then the ovaries develop from the cortex and the testes develop from the medulla of the gonad embryonic tissue. Look at Figure 21-6 in the textbook to see how the undifferentiated external genitalia develop into fully differential structures.

Organs of Reproduction

The female reproductive system includes two ovaries, two fallopian tubes, one uterus, and one vagina. The male reproductive system includes two testes, seminal ducts, glands, and the penis.

Female Reproductive System.

Ovaries.   Ovaries are the primary sex organs of the female; they produce germ cells and the hormones estrogen and progesterone.

> *Graafian follicle:* each ovary contains thousands of follicles, which when influenced by FSH of the pituitary are responsible for the process of the development of the ova into mature ova. The follicles also produce estrogen.
>
> *Ovulation:* the follicle enlarges, migrates to the outside of the ovary, and breaks open, releasing the ovum from the ovary.
>
> *Corpus luteum:* name given to the ruptured graafian follicle after ovulation; these cells produce progesterone.

Fallopian Tubes.   Fallopian tubes, or oviducts, are attached at one end to the uterus; the other end curves over the ovary. Its fimbriated ends catch the ovum when ovulation occurs. The tubes propel the ova down the tube to the uterus.

Uterus.   The uterus is a muscular organ that can greatly expand to accommodate a fetus. It is divided into three parts:

> *Fundus:* bulging, rounded, upper part
>
> *Body:* middle part of the uterus
>
> *Cervix:* lower, narrow portion that extends into the vagina

The **uterine wall** is three layers, the outer serous layer, or *visceral;* the middle muscular layer, the *myometrium;* and the inner mucous layer, the *endometrium,* which changes in consistency each month.

Vagina.   The vagina is the short canal that extends from the cervix of the uterus to the vulva. The *hymen* is a semipermeable membrane found at the entrance to the vagina.

External Female Genitalia.   The external female genitalia, or *vulva,* contains the external organs of the reproductive system.

> *Mons pubis:* a mound of fatty tissue over the pubic bone, covered with coarse hair
>
> *Vestibule:* area surrounding the openings of the urethra and the vagina
>
> *Clitoris:* small structure above the urethral opening, contains many nerve endings
>
> *Labia majora* and *labia minora:* folds of skin surrounding the vagina
>
> *Bartholin's glands:* mucous glands at the entrance to the vagina
>
> *Perineum:* area between the vagina and the rectum

Breasts.   Breasts are accessory organs of the reproductive system. They produce milk after childbirth. The *areola* is the dark area that surrounds the nipple.

Menstrual Cycle.   In the menstrual cycle, a mature egg develops and is ovulated every 28 days, beginning at puberty. The menstrual cycle is divided into four stages: follicle, ovulation, corpus luteum, and menstruation.

In the **follicle stage,** FSH secreted from the pituitary gland stimulates a graafian follicle in the ovary. The follicle grows, producing *estrogen,* and the egg cell matures. Estrogen stimulates the endometrium lining and is necessary for secondary sex characteristics. The follicle stage lasts 10 days.

In the **ovulation stage,** the estrogen blood level rises and the pituitary stops producing FSH and starts producing LH. The combination of hormone activity causes the follicle to rupture, and a mature ovum is released (*ovulation*). The ovulation stage occurs around the fourteenth day of the cycle.

In the **corpus luteum stage,** after ovulation, LH stimulates the graafian cells to change to cells called the *corpus luteum,* which produce *progesterone.* This hormone maintains the growth of the endometrium and inhibits FSH; this stage lasts 14 days.

In the **menstruation stage,** if fertilization does not occur, the progesterone level rises, inhibiting the LH hormone. As LH drops, the corpus luteum disintegrates and the lining of the endometrium breaks down and is discharged through the vagina. *Menstruation* has occurred. See Figure 21-12 in your textbook. Menstruation occurs and the estrogen level drops, causing FSH from the pituitary to start the cycle again.

Menopause is the time in a female's life when the menstrual cycle ceases; it occurs between 45 and 55 years of age. Physiological changes occur in the reproductive organs. "Hot flashes" and some psychological changes may also occur.

Male Reproductive System.

Testes.   Testes are the primary male reproductive organs. They lie outside the body in the *scrotum* (an external sac). They produce sperm and testosterone and are divided into partitions or lobules.

> **Seminiferous tubules** are found in each lobule; FSH stimulates the production of *sperm* in cells that line the tubules.
>
> *Interstitial tissue* supports the seminiferous tubules. The cells produce *testosterone,* necessary for growth and development of reproductive organs and secondary sex characteristics.

In the descent of the **testicles,** the testes, which develop in the abdominal cavity, in the last 3 months of embryonic life move downward into the scrotum. If the testes do not descend, the condition is known as *cryptorchidism.* This condition must be corrected, or spermatogenesis will not occur.

Epididymides.   The epididymides are overlying structures to which the testes are attached. They are formed by networks of seminiferous tubules.

Ductus Deferens, Seminal Vesicles, and Ejaculatory Ducts.   *Ductus deferens* or *vas deferens* are a continuation of the epididymis; they serve as storage sites for sperm cells and excretory ducts of the testes. The vas deferens enter the abdominal cavity in the inguinal area, wrap around the bladder, and meet the seminal vesicles. *Seminal vesicles* are two highly convoluted membranous tubes that produce seminal fluid, which is added to the sperm cells. *Ejaculatory ducts* are formed by the vas deferens and the seminal vesicles. They descend into the prostate gland to join with the urethra.

Penis.   The penis is the external organ of the male reproductive system. It contains erectile tissue. The *foreskin* is the loose-fitting skin that covers the end of the penis. *Circumcision* is a procedure in which the foreskin is removed.

Prostate Gland.   The prostate gland is located under the urinary bladder. It surrounds the opening of the bladder leading to the urethra and secretes a fluid that enhances sperm mobility.

Bulbourethral or Cowper's Glands.   The bulbourethral or Cowper's glands are located on either side of the urethra below the prostate gland; they add an alkaline fluid to semen.

Erection and Ejaculation.   When the male is sexually aroused, nerve impulses cause the erectile tissue to engorge with blood, which makes the tissue increase in size and become firm. Stimulating the glans penis results in stimulation of the seminal vesicles, impulses are sent to the ejaculatory center, and orgasm occurs. Secretions stored in the vas deferens, ejaculatory ducts, and prostate gland are forcibly expelled through the urethra and the engorgement ceases.

Impotence.   Impotence is the inability to have or sustain an erection. *Primary* impotence is when the male has never had an erection. *Secondary* impotence is current impotence. Transient periods of impotence are not a dysfunction. The cause of impotence is mostly organic; treatment includes penile implants, injections, and oral medications.

Contraception

Contraception is the conscious decision not to reproduce. Abstinence, a healthy choice, is voluntarily refraining from intercourse. See Table 21-4 in your textbook for other methods of contraception.

Infertility

Infertility is the inability to reproduce. Causes may be damage to the fallopian tubes, low sperm count, hormonal imbalance, and other disorders. Treatments include the following:

Fertility drugs promote ovulation by stimulating hormones.

Artificial insemination involves placing semen into the vaginal canal by a cannula and syringe around the time of ovulation.

Surgery to open blocked tube is called laparoscopy.

Assisted Reproductive Techniques include the following:

In vitro fertilization is ovulation-inducing drugs stimulate the development of multiple ovarian follicles. A laparoscopy is done to remove the follicles and extract the ova. The ova are cultured in vitro with sperm; if fertilization is successful, the zygote at the four- to eight-cell stage is transferred to the uterus.

Gamete intrafallopian tube transfer is the zygote is transferred into the end of the fallopian tube.

Effects of Aging

Hormone production declines and there may be atrophic changes. In the female, menopause occurs; in the male, changes are more gradual.

Disorders of the Female Reproductive System

Amenorrhea: absence of menstruation, normal in pregnancy

Dysmenorrhea: painful menstruation

Premenstrual syndrome (PMS): symptoms exhibited just before the menstrual cycle

Leukorrhea: whitish discharge from the vagina

Fibroid tumors: benign growths that occur in the uterine wall

Endometriosis: endometrial tissue outside the uterine cavity. The tissue responds to hormonal changes. Tissue outside the uterus allows no way for the blood to leave the body, resulting in internal bleeding, inflammation, and pain

Breast cancer: the most common cancer in women. Early detection is critical. Women should do breast self-exams, as well as have annual *mammograms* after the age of 40

Endometrial cancer: usually occurs after menopause

Ovarian cancer: leading cause of cancer death in women between the ages of 40 to 65

Cervical cancer: can be detected by a *Pap smear,* which is a sample of cell scrapings of the cervix and cervical canal

Infections of the Female Reproductive Organs.

Pelvic inflammatory disease (PID): infection that occurs in the reproductive organs and spreads to the fallopian tubes and peritoneal cavity. It is treated with antibiotics

Salpingitis: inflammation of the fallopian tubes

Toxic shock syndrome: bacterial infection, by the organism *Staphylococcus.*

Vaginal yeast infection: caused by fungus; symptoms are itching, burning, redness, and leukorrhea

Male Reproductive Disorders.

Epididymitis: painful swelling in the groin and scrotum caused by infection

Orchitis: infection of the testes; complication of mumps

Prostatitis: infection of the prostate gland

Benign prostatic hypertrophy (BPH): indicates an enlarged prostate, which occurs in most men after the age of 70; urinary problems develop

Prostate cancer: most common cancer in men after the age of 50. Males over age 40 should have annual rectal exams as well as a prostate specific antigen blood screening test, which detects an abnormal substance released by the cancer cells

Sexually Transmitted Diseases

Sexually transmitted diseases (STDs) are also known as *venereal diseases.* They are transmitted through the exchange of body fluids, such as semen, vaginal fluid, and blood. The most common are chlamydia, genital herpes, and genital warts. Protection from STDs includes abstinence and practicing safe sexual behavior. All STDs must be treated, because they may lead to sterility in females.

Chlamydia is the major cause of urethritis, bacterial vaginitis, and PID. Up to 80% of affected women and 25% of men have no symptoms.

Genital warts can appear on the shaft of the penis or inside the vagina. The disease may be asymptomatic; diagnosis is made by examination.

Genital herpes is a viral infection; blisterlike areas may appear on genitalia and cause a burning sensation. Symptoms may disappear after 2 weeks, but may reappear throughout the lifetime.

Gonorrhea is a bacterial infection. Males have painful urination and a discharge of pus from the penis; females may be asymptomatic. It is treated with antibiotics.

Syphilis is a bacterial sexually transmitted disease, treated with antibiotics.

Trichomoniasis vaginalis infection is caused by protozoan treated with antibiotics.

ACTIVITIES

A.   Describe the functions of the reproductive system.

_____

_____

_____

_____

_____

B.   Select the letter of the choice that best completes the statement.

1. The specialized sex cells or germ cells are also known as:
   a. gonads
   b. testicles
   c. ovaries
   d. gametes

2. In the formation of the germ cells, the specialized cell division process is known as:
   a. mitosis
   b. spermatogenesis
   c. meiosis
   d. oogenesis

3. In the male there is one pair of single sex chromosomes, an X and a Y, and:
   a. 22 autosomal pairs
   b. 22 autosomal single chromosomes
   c. 23 autosomal pairs
   d. 23 autosomal single chromosomes

4. Spermatozoa entering the female reproductive tract live for:
   a. 1 to 2 days
   b. 2 to 3 days
   c. 3 to 4 days
   d. 1 week

5. In one ejaculation, 100 million sperm may be deposited in 1 ml of seminal fluid. A person is considered sterile if the count is less than:
   a. 10 million per milliliter
   b. 20 million per milliliter
   c. 30 million per milliliter
   d. 40 million per milliliter

6. Sperm may die before they can approach the ovum for all of the following reasons except:
   a. high temperature of the female abdomen
   b. high acidity of the secretions in the vagina
   c. specialized lining of the uterus
   d. lack of the propulsion ability

7. For fertilization to occur, the layer of epithelial cells must fall away from the ovum. This layer is called:
   a. corona radiata
   b. zona pellucida
   c. hyaluronidase
   d. hyaluronic acid

8. True fertilization occurs when the sperm nucleus and the egg nucleus unite for a fertilized egg cell or:
   a. gamete
   b. gonad
   c. zygote
   d. embryo

9. The early process of cell division whereby the fertilized cell repeatedly divides and redivides is known as:
   a. fetus
   b. zygote
   c. cleavage
   d. gamete

10. The gender of the child is determined by:
    a. chromosome of the male parent
    b. chromosome of the female parent
    c. either male or female parent
    d. timing of pregnancy

C. Label the structure of the sperm and ovum. Color each structure.

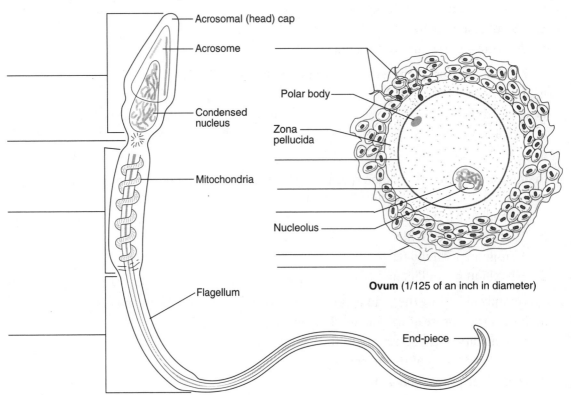

Ovum (1/125 of an inch in diameter)

D. Complete the following statements regarding male and female differences.

1. For the first 2 months, the embryo develops without a _____ identity.

2. The gonads of the female begin to evolve at or about the _____ or _____ week of pregnancy.

3. The ovaries of the female evolve from the _____ of the gonad, while the testes of the male evolve from the _____ of the gonad.

4. Internally the embryonic Wolffian ducts become the _____, _____, _____ and _____ _____ in the male.

5. Internally, the embryonic muellerian ducts become the _____, _____, _____, and the upper portion of the _____ in the female.

E. The undifferentiated external genitalia develop into fully differentiated structures. Complete the following statements.

In the male:

1. The tubercle becomes the _____ _____.

2. The folds become the _____ _____.

3. The swelling becomes the _____.

In the female:

1. The tubercle becomes the _____.

2. The folds become the _____ _____.

3. The swelling becomes the _____ _____.

F. Label the female organs of reproduction. Color the uterus layers red, brown, and orange; the fallopian tubes yellow; the ovaries pink, the fungus red; and the vagina pink.

Ovarian ligament

E. _____

Infundibulum _____

Uterine cavity _____

F. _____

G. _____

H. _____

D.

C.

B.

Cervix

A.

G.   Match the letters on the previous diagram with the following descriptions.

_____   1. Produce ova and the hormones estrogen and progesterone

_____   2. Oviducts, carry the ova to the uterus

_____   3. Smooth, muscular layer of the uterus

_____   4. Inner mucous layer of the uterus

_____   5. Short canal that extends from the cervix to the vulva

_____   6. Bulging, rounded part of the uterus

_____   7. Canal that extends from the lower uterine cavity to the external os at the end of the cervix

_____   8. Outer end of the oviduct that curves over the top edge of each ovary

H.   Name three functions each of estrogen and progesterone.

_____

_____

_____

_____

_____

_____

I.   Mark the following statements as either true or false. Correct any false statements.

_____   1. The reproductive years begin at the time of puberty and menarche.

_____   2. Fertilization of the ovum takes place in the inner third of the oviduct.

_____   3. The hymen found at or near the entrance to the vaginal canal has some openings that allow for the menstrual flow.

_____   4. The external female genital is also called the vulva.

_____   5. The area surrounding the urethra and the vagina is called the vestibule, and the urethra is inferior to the vagina.

_____   6. Above the urethral opening is the clitoris, which contains many nerve endings.

_____   7. The perineum is the area between the vaginal opening and the rectum; it consists of muscles that form a sphincter for the vulva.

_____   8. During childbirth, a surgical opening into the perineum is called an episiotomy.

_____   9. The area surrounding the nipple is called the areola.

_____ 10. Prolactin from the posterior lobe of the pituitary gland stimulates the mammary glands to secrete milk following childbirth.

J. Select the appropriate word or words about the menstrual cycle from the following list to complete the statements. A word may be used more than once.

corpus luteum	decreasing	discharged	endometrium
estrogen	FSH	fallopian tube	follicle
follicles	implantation	LH	menstruation
one	ovaries	ovulation	pituitary
progesterone	puberty	ruptures	uterine
4	5	9	10
12	14	15	17

1. The menstrual cycle starts at _____ and begins as early as _____ years of age or as late as _____ years of age. Generally, the age is between _____ and _____.

2. Changes that occur during the menstrual cycle involve hormones from the _____ gland and the _____.

3. The four stages of the menstrual cycle are _____, _____, _____, and _____.

4. _____ from the _____ gland is secreted on day 5 of the cycle.

5. It reaches the ovary through the bloodstream and stimulates several _____; however, only _____ matures.

6. As the follicle grows, an egg cell develops inside, and the follicle fills with a fluid containing _____.

7. The _____ stimulates the _____ to thicken with mucus and a rich supply of blood vessels to prepare the endometrium for the _____ of a fertilized egg.

8. The follicle stage lasts _____ days.

9. When the _____ level increases in the blood, the pituitary stops secreting _____.

10. The _____ hormone is now secreted by the pituitary.

11. The three hormones circulating in the blood at this time are _____, _____, and _____ in different concentrations.

12. On day 14 this combination stimulates the mature follicle to _____, releasing the egg into the _____ _____.

13. This event is called _____.

14. After _____, LH stimulates the cells of the ruptured follicle to divide quickly; this mass of cells is now called the _____ _____.

15. The _____ _____ produces a hormone called _____, which maintains the growth of the endometrium.

16. Progesterone inhibits the release of _____.

17. The corpus luteum stage lasts about _____ days.

18. If fertilization does not occur, the progesterone reaches a level in the bloodstream that inhibits _____ secretion from the pituitary.

19. With the drop in LH, the corpus luteum breaks down _____ progesterone levels.

20. As the progesterone level decreases, the endometrial lining breaks away from the _____ wall and is _____ from the body with the unfertilized egg.

21. This is the menstrual stage and lasts about _____ days.

22. The estrogen level is also _____ at this time, which then stimulates the pituitary to secrete _____ and the cycle begins again.

23. The first day of the menstrual cycle begins with the_____ day of menstruation.

K. Label the ovary, showing the development of the graafian follicle.

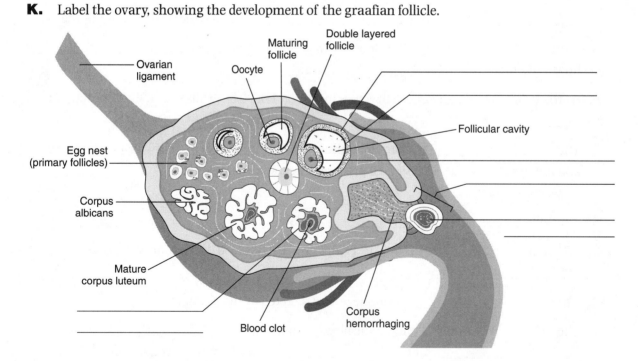

L. Answer the following questions about menopause.

 1. Define menopause.

    _____

    _____

2. Describe the anatomical changes that occur during menopause.

_____

_____

_____

3. Describe the physiological changes that occur during menopause.

_____

_____

_____

4. Describe the psychological changes that occur during menopause.

_____

_____

_____

_____

M. Label the male reproductive system. Color the vas deferens and continuing structures brown from where it starts in the testes to the penis.

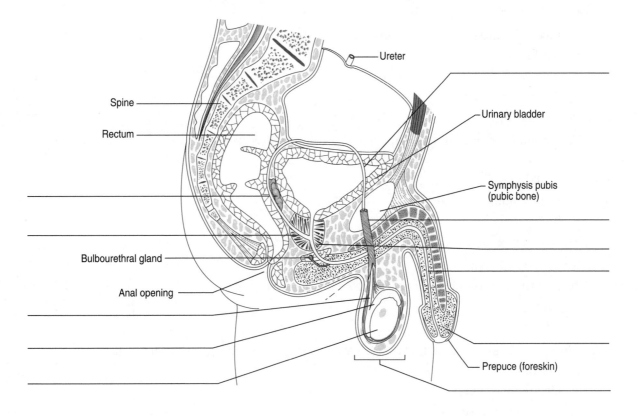

N. Select the letter of the choice that best completes the statement.

1. The testes produce the male gametes and the male hormone testosterone; they are encased in a pouch called the:
   a. testicular
   b. epididymis
   c. scrotum
   d. seminal ducts

2. The pathway of sperm is through a series of ducts from the:
   a. epididymis, seminal ducts, ejaculatory ducts, and urethra
   b. epididymis, ejaculatory ducts, seminal ducts, and urethra
   c. seminal ducts, epididymis, ejaculatory ducts, and urethra
   d. epididymis, urethra, seminal ducts, and ejaculatory ducts

3. The testes are attached to an overlying structure called the:
   a. epididymis
   b. tunica albuginea
   c. lobule
   d. seminiferous tubules

4. Each testicular lobule contains seminiferous tubules that produce sperm under the influence of:
   a. LH
   b. FSH
   c. ICSH
   d. testosterone

5. In males, mature sperm formation requires about:
   a. 50 days
   b. 28 days
   c. 7 days
   d. 24 days

6. The seminiferous tubules are supported by tissue, which produces testosterone, called:
   a. rete testis
   b. epididymis
   c. tunica albuginea
   d. interstitial

7. The vas deferens are continuations of the:
   a. interstitial tissue
   b. seminiferous tubules
   c. epididymis
   d. rete testis

8. The seminal vesicle has a duct that leads away from it to join the vas deferens and form the:
   a. urethra
   b. ejaculatory duct
   c. prostatic urethra
   d. penis

9. The ejaculatory ducts descend into the prostrate gland to join with the:
   a. penis
   b. ureter
   c. urethra
   d. prepuce

10. The prostate gland is located:
    a. superior to the bladder
    b. inferior to the bladder
    c. posterior to the rectum
    d. lateral to the rectum

O. Answer the following questions relating to the reproductive system.

1. Describe the function of the prostate gland.

   _____

   _____

   _____

2. Describe the location and function of the bulbourethral glands.

   _____

   _____

   _____

3. How does ejaculation occur?

   _____

   _____

4. Define primary and secondary impotence.

   _____

   _____

   _____

5. What is the treatment for impotence?

   _____

   _____

6. Define contraception.

   _____

   _____

7. Give several reasons to avoid conception.

_____

_____

8. Define infertility.

_____

_____

P. Circle the correctly spelled word in each of the following statements.

1. (Amenorhea, Amenorrhea) is a term used to define absence of (menstruation, menstuation).

2. Dysmenorrhea is characterized by cramps that may be caused by excessive production of (prostaglandin, prostoglandin).

3. Endometrial tissue is found outside the uterus in the condition known as (endometrisis, endometriosis).

4. Benign tumors of the uterus are known as (fibroids, fiboids).

5. Breast cancer can be detected in its early stage if women have routine mammograms and do breast exams by (palpating, palpatating) their breasts.

6. A mammogram is recommended on an (anuall, annual) basis for all women over the age of 40.

7. To treat fibroids or endometrial cancer, a (hysterectomy, histerectomy) may be done.

8. (Cervical, Cervixal) cancer is seen in women between the ages of 30 and 50.

9. To diagnose cancer of the cervix, a (Papinacolaou, Papanicolaou) smear is done.

10. A (laporoscopy, laparoscopy) is a minor surgical procedure in which the patient's abdomen is distended with carbon dioxide gas; an instrument, the (laporscope, laparoscope) is inserted (thorugh, through) a tiny incision into the abdomen.

Q. Match the disorder in Column A with the statement describing it in Column B.

Column A	Column B
_____ 1. pelvic inflammatory disease	a. itching, burning of the vulva
_____ 2. toxic shock syndrome	b. inflammation of the fallopian tubes
_____ 3. salpingitis	c. infection of the reproductive organs
_____ 4. vaginal yeast infection	d. infection caused by staphylococcus

R. Mark the following statements as either true or false. Correct any false statements.

_____ 1. A painful swelling in the groin and scrotum is epididymitis.

_____ 2. An inflammation of the testes is testitis.

_____ 3. An inflammation of the prostate gland is prostatitis.

_____ 4. The most common cancer in men over the age of 50 is lung cancer; another common cancer is prostate cancer.

_____ 5. The most common treatment for prostate cancer is prostatectomy.

S. Answer the following questions about sexually transmitted diseases.

1. Define what is meant by the term *sexually transmitted disease (STD)*.

_____

_____

_____

2. Describe some of symptoms of STD that may occur.

_____

_____

_____

3. Explain how to prevent STD.

_____

_____

_____

T. Use the words from the following list to complete the story about reproduction.

abdominal	endometrium	seminal vesicles
alkaline	cervix	testicular
bladder	fertilization	urethra
Cowper's gland	fallopian tube	vagina
ductus deferens	egg	uterus
epididymis	sperm	

THE BEGINNING OF LIFE

I was waiting and waiting to start a new life;
it finally happened when my host married a wife.

I started out life in a _____ cell,
and became a mature _____ in a place called the _____ dell.

I left this long and tubelike place,
and traveled up the _____ _____ into the _____ space.

I was shipped around the _____ head, neck, and tail.
and squirted with fluid that made me hearty and hale.

First came fluid from the _____ ; _____
it was the first big drink since I left the testicle.

The tunnel I traveled went through a tight spot,

the prostatic _____, where I received another _____ pop.

I'm now ready to leave, but before I go—

_____ _____ gives me an alkaline bath to make me fast not slow.

I couple with the host's new wife;

they are both eager to begin a new life.

I squeeze up through the _____, a muscular tube,

and enter the _____, pretty well lubed.

I swim up the _____, which is shaped like a balloon,

taking a look at the place I hope to move into soon.

The _____ lining is thick in preparation

to receive me and the ovum after _____.

I move to a _____ _____ and see an _____ shining bright;

which I know I will be able to penetrate tonight.

This is wonderful: We two have become one.

And now our new life has begun.

APPLYING THEORY TO PRACTICE

1. Rebecca, age 13, questions her mother regarding menstruation. She is concerned her body will look different. Her mother explains to Rebecca some of the physical and emotional changes that will occur when menstruation starts. List the changes that will occur.

   _____

   _____

   _____

2. Tanya is a 36-year-old mother who has a family history of breast cancer. Both her mother and grandmother had breast cancer. She has been doing self breast exams and now hears that this may not be an effective way to detect breast tumors. Tanya questions Keisha, the medical assistant, regarding this topic. Tanya also wants information on the new recommended treatment for breast cancer.

   _____

   _____

   _____

3. Leslie has severe cramping during her menstrual cycles. After taking a health history and an examination, a diagnosis of endometriosis is made. What information can Nichole, the nurse at the women's health center, give to Leslie on endometriosis and effective treatment for this condition?

_____

_____

_____

4. Some men are afraid of having a physical examination for BPH or prostate cancer. They fear that the treatment for these conditions will cause impotence. Dr. Joseph, a urologist, is concerned that men will not be checked for prostate cancer because of this fear. He is asked to address a group of local businessmen and discuss this topic. What information can Dr. Joseph give to the group?

_____

_____

_____

5. Sexually transmitted diseases are increasing in number. You are asked to participate in a panel discussion in your school regarding this problem. In addition to knowing the cause and the treatment, what other types of advice can you give to prevent this problem? Include in your discussion chlamydia, genital warts, gonorrhea, genital herpes, and syphilis.

_____

_____

_____

_____

_____

_____

_____

_____

SURF THE NET

Briefly summarize your findings from the suggested Web sites, or choose alternate sites for the following:

1. To study the female reproductive system, go to
   http://www.gen_umn.edu/faculty_staff/jensen/1135/webanatomy/wa

2. To see how a baby grows (fetal development), go to http://www.babycenter.com/fetal

3. For information on fertility problems, go to http://www.babycenter.com/refcap/4089.html

4. Search for Web sites with additional information on sexually transmitted diseases.

Genetics and Genetically Linked Diseases

OVERVIEW

Genetics is the branch of biology that studies how the genes are transmitted from parents to offspring.

Chromosomes are the structures found in the nucleus of each germ cell that contain DNA.

A **gene** is a small unit of DNA found along the length of the chromosome. It carries information for the cellular synthesis of a specific protein.

Mutations are the appearances of new and different traits caused by changes in the chromosome. Types of mutation include the following:

Gene mutation: a new or altered gene is produced to replace a normal or preexisting gene.

Chromosomal mutation: change in the number of chromosomes found in the nucleus or a change in the structure of a whole chromosome.

Types of gene mutation include the following:

Somatic cell: mutation that occurs in individual body (somatic) cells. It is not inherited (e.g., skin changes as we age).

Gametic cell: mutation that occurs in the nucleus of the germ cells that will be passed to the next generation.

Lethal gene: results in death in utero or later in life.

Human Genetic Disorders

A **genetic disorder** or **hereditary disorder** is caused by a variation in the genetic pattern, whereas a *congenital disorder* evolves during fetal development and is not related to a genetic malformation.

Phenylketonuria (PKU): human metabolic disorder, caused by an enzyme deficiency, where amino acids cannot break down causing mental retardation.

Sickle cell anemia: abnormal hemoglobin molecule in red blood cell; common in individuals of African descent.

Tay-Sachs disease: deficiency of a lysosomal enzyme which breaks down fat; the fat molecules then accumulate in the brain cells and destroy them.

Huntington's disease: degeneration of the central nervous system.

Duchenne's muscular dystrophy: muscles suffer loss of protein and the contractile fibers are eventually replaced by fat and connective tissue, rendering the skeletal muscles useless.

Cystic fibrosis: lining of the digestive tract, ducts of the pancreas, and the respiratory tract produce thick mucus which blocks the passageways.

Thalassemia (Cooley's anemia): blood disorder found in people of Mediterranean descent.

Hemophilia: sex-linked disorder; person is unable to produce the factor VIII which is necessary for blood clotting; mothers can pass this disease to sons.

Chromosomal Aberrations.   *Down's syndrome (mongolism)* involves an extra chromosome designated as chromosome 21. *Mutagenic agents* speed up the occurrence of mutations.

Genetic Counseling.   *Genetic counseling* involves talking with parents or prospective parents about the possibility of genetic disorders.

Genetic Testing.   Genetic testing may be diagnostic tests done during pregnancy to determine genetic problems.

Amniocentesis is the withdrawal of amniotic fluid during week 16 of pregnancy which can pick up as many as 200 possible genetic disorders.

Chorionic villi sampling may be done as early as 8 to 10 weeks into the pregnancy; a sample of fetal cells is removed from the fetal side of the placenta.

Genetic engineering is gene transfer from the cell of one species to another or isolating a specific gene and growing copies of it. An example of genetic engineering is interferon.

Interferon are proteins that interfere with virus replication using the sophisticated technology of recombinant DNA which alters gene structure.

ACTIVITIES

A.   Use the words from the following list to complete the statements. Words may be used more than once.

childhood	embryology	mitosis	synthesis
chromosomes	fertilization	mutation	teens
chromosomal	gene	recessive	adulthood
DNA	genetics	RNA	reproductive
dominant	lethal	somatic cell	

1.   The process by which an egg and a sperm unite is called _____.

2.   A gene is an area of _____ that carries information for the cellular _____ of a specific protein.

3.   Due to the combined influence of all the genes on all the _____, a new individual is formed.

4.   The branch of biology that studies how genes are transmitted from parents to child is _____.

5.   The inheritance of a changed or mutated gene will cause the appearance of a new and different trait called a _____.

6. When a new or altered gene is produced to replace a preexisting gene it is called
   _____ mutation; when there is a change in the number of chromosomes, it
   is a _____ mutation.

7. Mutations that occur but will not be transmitted to offspring, such as how the skin changes as
   we age, are called _____ _____ mutations.

8. A gene that results in death is called a _____ gene. It may occur during
   embryonic development or later in life.

9. Most persons carry two to three _____ genes; two similar
   _____ genes must be present in an individual for the gene to be expressed.

10. Lethal genes that exert their influence later in life are Tay-Sachs disease (death occurs during
    _____ years), Duchenne's muscular dystrophy (death usually occurs during
    or _____ years), and Huntington's disease (death occurs during
    _____ years).

B. Select the letter of the choice that best completes the statement.

1. A genetic disorder is caused by:
   a. a condition that occurs in the first trimester
   b. a condition that occurs during delivery
   c. a condition that occurs in the last trimester
   d. a condition caused by a variation in the genetic pattern

2. PKU is caused by an enzyme deficiency in which:
   a. the red blood cell forms a sickle shape
   b. lipids accumulate in the brain
   c. amino acids build up in the brain
   d. muscles atrophy

3. The test done at birth is for the genetic disorder:
   a. PKU
   b. sickle cell anemia
   c. Huntington's disease
   d. Down syndrome

4. The enzyme missing in this disorder causes lipid molecules to accumulate in the brain:
   a. Tay-Sachs disease
   b. cystic fibrosis
   c. hemophilia
   d. PKU

5. Degeneration of the central nervous system occurs in:
   a. Tay-Sachs disease
   b. cystic fibrosis
   c. thalassemia minor
   d. Huntington's disease

6. Duchenne's muscular dystrophy affects the:
    a. contractile fibers of skeletal muscle
    b. respiratory passages, which become thick with mucus
    c. smooth muscle of the digestive tract
    d. limbs, causing spastic paralysis

7. In cystic fibrosis, the linings of exocrine glands become filled with mucous plugs. The system most affected is the:
    a. muscular system
    b. circulatory system
    c. digestive system
    d. central nervous system

8. Cupping and clapping is the treatment of choice for:
    a. Huntington's disease
    b. Tay-Sachs disease
    c. cystic fibrosis
    d. Down syndrome

9. In Down syndrome, the chromosomal aberration that occurs is:
    a. a pair of chromosomes adhering to each other
    b. a chromosome missing
    c. nondisjunction of sex chromosomes
    d. an extra chromosome

10. When a cell or group of cells is exposed to radiation or chemicals, the speed of mutation:
    a. is not affected
    b. increases
    c. decreases
    d. depends on the age of the individual

C. Answer the following questions.

1. In sickle cell anemia, what does the rapid destruction of sickle cells cause?

_____

2. Clumping of red blood cells causes damage to what systems of the body? What is the resulting disorder?

_____

_____

3. Name two genetic disorders that involve the red blood cells.

_____

_____

4. Name three genetic disorders that involve the central nervous system.

_____

_____

_____

5. Describe three tests done during genetic counseling.

_____

_____

_____

APPLYING THEORY TO PRACTICE

1. Name three genetic engineering products that use the technology of recombinant DNA.

_____

_____

_____

2. Describe gene therapy. List the people who may be especially interested in this topic.

_____

_____

_____

SURF THE NET

Briefly summarize your findings from the suggested Web sites, or choose alternate sites for the following topics.

1. For information on genetic disorders, go to
   http://www.noah-health.org/english/illness/genetic_diseases/geneticdis.html

2. For updates regarding genetic therapy, go to
   http://www-ermm.cbcu.cam.ac.uk/99000691h.htm